THE WELL WOMAN

A Journey to Wellness Through Loving Jesus

GENA ANDERSON

CONTENTS

ACKNOWLEDGMENTS

To my husband, thank you for believing in, supporting, and loving me through the writing of this work, and always. I'm blessed by you every day. Thank you to my kids, for bringing me joy. To Luke, thank you for marketing my book to your teachers and the Hutto Public Library, I love your complete faith in me and your heart. And to my Jocelyn, may this work reflect even an ounce of the beauty and light you bring to this world and my life.

To my parents, and the people they put in my lives to influence my early years, thank you for molding this quiet girl into the woman who could write this work.

To the Created Woman Family, and our fearless leader Heather, thank you for empowering me to be who I was created to be and being a constant source of support and friendship. Martha, thank you for your diligence in editing my work and teaching me with kindness.

To Heather Bise, your wise and gentle guidance was the catalyst that took this book from idea to a written work, and I am forever grateful.

To my lifelong friends, Naomi, Lexy, Mindy, and Jessica, I am so glad you're in my corner, and I treasure your support in life and with this book.

To Deb Hall, this book would be a riddled with unnecessary words, misplaced commas, and generally a poorly formatted mess without you, and I thank you for going above and beyond.

To Stephanie Yttrup, thank you for your patience and creativity in drafting a beautiful cover.

To Meghan Hendry, you are wise beyond your years and I cherish your friendship and thank you for so graciously helping me.

And, to all my family and friends who have cheered for and encouraged me, I cannot thank you enough. There are more names than there are lines on this page. I have not forgotten, could not forget, each one who has been a part of my journey to this point. I am eternally grateful to each soul who has poured into my life what I'm now able to pour out into the world.

INTRODUCTION

I can tell we have much in common, you and I. The first clue? You are holding this book in your hands and reading these words. That tells me you are either my mom, a sweet, supportive friend, or someone who also struggles to achieve and maintain true wellness, not just good health. If you opened this book, which clearly you did, I know you not only want to be well, but you're actively seeking the solution to your wellness woes. If I could sit down with you, I'd listen to your story, your desires for your life and health, the things you've tried successfully and the failed attempts, and the things you haven't overcome. I might offer some friendly advice, an empathetic nod, and a little encouragement, but I'd want to give you exponentially more.

Friend, there is a reason you hold this book in your hands. It is the culmination of wisdom I've gained thus far on the topic of wellness, and it is the message of healthy hope God has given me to share with you. It's my gift to you, and it's so much more than I could offer in one conversation. As you unwrap this gift, chapter by chapter, I pray you receive what every good gift should offer: something you desperately desire for yourself but haven't yet obtained. The gift of wellness awaits, and I'm honored to walk you through the journey of finding it.

You'd probably like to know a bit about me. I'm a wife, mom, and professional whose days are filled with work, kids' activities, and all the things required to keep a home with four people and three dogs running. What would inspire me to carve out time from the flurries of life and write this labor of love? The answer is simple. I've witnessed firsthand, while simultaneously building my own knowledge on the topic, the abundant need in women for wellness. The combination of an evolving awareness of this devastating problem along with a recognition of the solution both broke my heart and gave me hope for women. The more aware I became, the more I became compelled to get this message out, in writing, to the women of this world.

I work as a family nurse practitioner. The title of this book was birthed out of my desire to inspire wellness in women and my struggle to help women be well. A woman's annual physical is called a "well woman" visit. I wholeheartedly encourage annual checkups as a time to make sure you are connecting with your provider, taking a good overall look at your health, and screening for any conditions you may be at risk for developing. It's a proven way to prevent diseases or detect them early. However, a well woman exam, though highly beneficial, could not possibly address all the multifaceted and complex issues that make up the wellness of a woman. I often find, at the conclusion of this thorough and time-consuming visit, that we have only scratched the surface of true wellness. I know more can be done to help us feel our best and become what we were intended to become. I want more for my patients, myself, and you than the absence of disease. I want us to be well.

1 WHAT'S WELLNESS?

I'm going to come out and say it: I totally judge books by their covers. I should know better than most the monstrosity of time, effort, and investment it takes to write the words that fill the many pages of a book, yet I determine the quality by what I can most readily see. Don't we all do this? We make judgments based on what we can see, and we don't always consider the unseen. We share the perfectly posed Instagram photo of our dinner, leaving the rest of the messy kitchen out of the frame. Yet that woman who appears so beautifully put together on the outside may be withering away on the inside. There's always more to the story than the cover, and it's the stuff on the inside that reveals what the book, or the woman, is all about.

Wellness is like that. It inspires the outside but can't always be accurately determined by what's visible to the world around us. That's why this book is about working from the inside out, focusing on the inside first, giving every woman who reads it the opportunity to be transformed wholly and fully.

Before jumping into this pursuit of wellness, let's first define the concept of a well woman. Who is she, and what is she like? More importantly, what does a well woman have that you don't (yet)? These are excellent questions, so let's take a few minutes to consider her qualities, then you can decide for yourself whether you want to know more.

THE WELL WOMAN

The well woman . . .

Loves the Lord with her whole heart.

Loves others.

Loves herself.

Knows she is a daughter of the King.

Believes she is worthy of being loved.

Knows she is valuable to the Lord.

Acts according to what she knows.

Hears the Lord so loud and clear that the voices of her haters are simply background noise.

Is imperfect and gives her flaws to the Lord.

Is forgiven for her wrongs.

Seeks healing of her wounds and illnesses.

Accepts forgiveness and healing from her loving Father.

Is covered by the righteousness of God, through the gift of Jesus.

Has joy regardless of circumstances.

Is beautiful to behold.

Possesses purpose.

Walks the path God has already laid out for her.

Is uniquely qualified to do what God has put in her path.

Is present and purposeful every day.

Follows through with what the Lord convicts her to do.

Sees her health as both a blessing from and a gift to the Lord.

Commits to daily tasks to seek wellness.

Fills her mind, body, and soul with nourishment.

Allows her physical self to reflect the Holy Spirit inside her.

Bravely displays her scars as her testimony.

Is grateful for the body she has.

Is able.

Is grateful for the life she's been given.

Sees today as a gift.

Knows whose she is and who she is.

She is a well woman.

As I reread through the above description of a well woman, which I have cultivated as I've walked with the Lord, every fiber of my being wants to be her. It brings tears to my eyes. Tears in remembrance of where I've been and in gratitude for where I'm going. We are all a work in progress, and so is she. This well woman, she didn't become well on her own, and the process wasn't completed overnight nor with ease. In fact, she is still in the process of becoming well.

Between those lines above, I see my story. I see the shame I've carried for past mistakes, the feelings of unworthiness, and the self-criticism. I see the fear, doubt, and anxiety that have held me back. I feel the pressures of this world that are at best distracting and at worst absolutely destructive. I see the attempted attacks of Satan to use my unhealthy tendencies as tools against me. I also see the work of God in her and in me. I see a steady progression through seeking Jesus daily. I see hope that even I can be a well woman. That hope is why I've sought to know more, and I hope you do too.

I'm so thankful you're taking the time to read this book, and I encourage you to make the most of your efforts, starting with a prayer. Your journey to wellness starts now.

Lord, you are a good God who offers more goodness to us than we deserve. Open our hearts and minds to your voice as we read these pages. Help us to slow down and listen. Guide our thoughts and help us reflect and learn from the past. Give us hope as we plan for a future. Inspire healthy change in us. In your name we declare a transformation, that we will become well women. Amen.

2 FALLING IN LOVE

About a decade ago I did what many of us do: I made a big goal for the new year. I decided I was going to read the Bible, cover to cover, in one year. It was something I felt I needed to do, and I knew it would be good for me. So, I set out with my determined commitment, but it didn't take long for all that excited motivation to turn. The goal was lofty, and reading through the Old Testament was less than thrilling; eventually I could no longer will myself to keep going, and I quit.

Have you ever wondered why we start resolutions every new year only to forget about them by the end of the first month? Why do we make bad choices, of any kind, when we know very well what we're doing is not what we should do? I think the more pressing question for the topic at hand is this: if we all want to be healthy and well, why do we continue to make choices to our detriment?

It's a tough question to which I've given considerable thought. It's a question that stings a bit. I've gained and lost the same ten pounds more times than I can count. Patients continually come into my exam room and make the statement, "I know what I need to be doing. I've just got to do it." We all make bad choices, despite knowing better.

The answer to all of the above questions is the same: we do what we want to do. We will typically only oblige what we don't want to do for a little while. Eventually our nature is to revert back to doing what we want. In my failed attempt to read the Bible, motivation was a big problem. I was motivated by obligation, not a sincere desire to do what I was doing. Some years later, I was able to be successful with that same goal because my motivation was different.

Motivation is the driving force behind so much of what we do. Certainly, there are external factors and uncontrollable life circumstances we do not choose that impact our health and our ability to make good choices. We will take a deep dive into that in chapter 5. What I want us to focus on right now is what motivates us to make the choices we make and what would compel us to want to make better ones.

Maslow's hierarchy of needs is a concept that we nurses are all too familiar with.[i] This theory proposes we are motivated to meet our most basic physical and safety needs first, followed by the need for love and esteem, and once those are met, the primary motivation is the desire for self-actualization, or becoming what we are meant to become. This theory is relatable, and it helps us to understand why we do some of the things we do.

When we're hangry and cooking dinner on a busy Wednesday, it's hard to remember we love that child who is interrupting us by calling our name no less than fourteen times in the last fifteen seconds. When we aren't sure how we are going to pay the bills, it's hard to think about God's great big plan for our future. When we have unmet basic needs, it's very difficult to focus on relationships, and it's even more difficult to focus on becoming well in new ways. This theory is helpful, and certainly a good observation of human behavior, but I'm not entirely sure it takes all factors for motivation into consideration. In fact, I suspect our motivation doesn't have to progress in that exact order, because I've learned a bypass Mr. Maslow may not have considered.

When I was a child and young adult, being a Christian meant something entirely different to me than it does now. In my younger years I thought Christianity was this box that was trying to suppress me with rules and commands of dos and don'ts. Some of these commands, like not committing murder, I was fine with. Others, like not making anything more important than God, I wasn't so fond of. Because boys and fun and money and lots of other stuff were pretty darn important. So, for a long time, I knew Jesus died for me and had saved me from myself, but I didn't fully appreciate that gift for what it was, and I lived half in and half out of this Christian box.

Life marched on, and eventually I began to see God's goodness in my life and appreciate this gift of salvation more. I also started to see that God wasn't necessarily the ruler, commander, and prohibitor I had envisioned. As I learned more about how God loved me and wanted a relationship with me, I developed a desire to know more about him. The motivation for me at that time became the knowledge of and gratitude for his love for me. I became more involved at church, even opening my own Bible some! This was quite some time before my first attempt to read the entire Bible in one year, I'm not talking about anything that deep or committed. It was more like "a verse a day keeps Satan away." It was a start. I found myself praying more often, and I began to feel like I was figuring this Christian thing out. My box became more like a soft place to land and a comfort zone that felt less restricting and more safe, secure, and welcoming.

It was during this time when I was learning to know and accept God's love for me that I heard a song while driving that would start me on a journey that blew that box right up. That song, entitled "More Like Falling in Love" by Jason Gray, described Christianity as being more like falling in love than simply believing in something or someone.

I remember very clearly how I felt about the lyrics of that song. They puzzled me. Falling in love? What kind of Bible-beating Jesus freak would say that? I mean, I love God, he loves me, and I go to church and stuff, but falling in love is a bit much. I don't want to be a crazy church lady; I just want to be a good person who believes in God. Nothing wrong with that, right?

Well, after a long journey, I can confirm there *is* something wrong with a room-temperature, surface-deep, and misinformed relationship with my Creator. On this journey, I've walked with, run from, run to, surrendered to, cried out to, and rested in the arms of my God, and he has shown me exactly what this song is talking about. His Word clearly tells us that we are to love him with an all-consuming love. As Deuteronomy 6:5 tells us, "You shall love the Lord your God with all your heart, with all your soul, and with all your strength" (NKJV).

This verse and many others make it crystal clear we are to love God with everything we've got. For some of us, it takes a little while to figure out how to do that. The best way I know to help you understand why I eventually changed my tune and fell completely in love with Jesus is to tell you exactly how it happened.

You've already gotten the short version of the early relationship, when we were friends and getting to know each other. I was introduced to God in a wonderful Baptist church in my hometown. For all the preschool and children's ministry teachers and all the mamas out there, who are currently planting seeds in young hearts, please know your work is valuable. I so appreciate those who poured into me during my younger years, and I know those seeds, though dormant for a time, were the start of all that was to come so many years later.

Technically, God already knew me quite well during this courtship, so I suppose it was more about me getting to know him. We spent time together off and on, and looking back I see now how he was always pursuing me, even when I chose to ignore him. In any relationship, we can usually identify a moment or season when things began to shift, when we began to fall in love. For me and God, it started not long after I heard that song I referenced above.

I mentioned that, in the years leading up to hearing that song, I started to realize there is more to this idea of being a Christian than rules and regulations. I started to understand God's unconditional love for me and wanted to know more about that. I wanted more out of my faith.

Ephesians 3:20–21 says, "Now to Him who is able to do exceedingly abundantly above all that we ask or think, according to the power that works in us, to Him be glory in the church by Christ Jesus to all generations, forever and ever. Amen" (NKJV). I love this verse because it points out God's ability to surpass not only our expectations but our wildest dreams! I wanted more, but I had no idea what more was, and I most certainly underestimated what God could do and would do with me.

When I heard Jason's Gray's song and those words about falling in love with Jesus, I was just beginning to understand God's love for me and to accept the idea that he had more. What's more important is I began to realize he had more *for me.* There is a distinct difference. We will talk about breaking free from strongholds later, but it was a huge step forward in my relationship with God and my wellness journey to realize I am loved, known, and valuable to God. Me.

John 3:16 says God loves us so much that he gave his son for us, in order to give us life! "For God loved the world in this way: He gave his one and only Son, so that everyone who believes in him will not perish but have eternal life" (John 3:16 CSB). If you have any doubt about how this applies to you, pause here. I understand what it's like to doubt this. Our world can be so unloving that we begin to question the genuineness of any love offered to us. God not only talks the talk; he also shows us exactly how genuine he is with real action. You need to know that God loves you so much, he died for you, specifically. He sacrificed his son in your place out of nothing but love for *you.* You are so dearly loved. If you're not convinced, stick with me a little longer and I'll share how God sealed the deal with me.

Hearing that song brought to the forefront of my mind and heart an awareness that I was not falling in love with Jesus, and I started to wonder about that. Shortly after, my life got difficult, and God and I took things to a whole new level, one I would not have willingly gone to on my own. It all started with some challenges in my marriage. If you've been married for any amount of time, you can relate. My husband and I had gotten to a point where we were so distant from each other that we could hardly speak without arguing. I think it's safe to say we were both pretty miserable, despite the outward appearance of a happy middle-class family. As our relationship spiraled, so did our finances, which added a lovely amount of stress and anxiety to the existing misery. Thankfully, God began to work on us, and we started to lean on him to repair and restore things.

In the very beginning of this restoration effort, we found out my mother-in-law had cancer. Enter grief, anger, and many other emotions to add to the above misery, stress, and anxiety. We brought her to live with us and were happy to do so because we knew her days on this earth were limited. We wanted to be there for her and with her, and will always treasure those memories. That time in our lives was a bit like childbirth: painful, exhausting, yet sprinkled with joy. Oh, and if I haven't mentioned yet, I had taken a relatively new and challenging full-time job, enrolled in a graduate program, and was raising two little people who were five and one at the time. To this day, as I write this, I rarely talk about this time in our lives because I can't do it without tears. Our days were filled with raising children, working, caring for my mother-in-law, and trying to make the most of the time we had with her. My morning commutes, after dropping off the kids at day care, were the only times I had with God alone, and I made the most of those with music, prayers, and lots of tears.

I distinctly remember a day, right before my mother-in-law moved in, when I came home after being at work all day. I walked inside the house, tired from work and life and trying to hold together a hurting marriage, and said to myself, "This is the last thing we need. Why would God do this to us now?" Little did I know that God would actually answer that question, in time.

Through this season, I couldn't help but take note of God's very distinct presence in our lives and our days. Whenever we had a need, it was always met somehow, every single time. Family and friends showed up at the right times to help us out. When my mother-in-law did leave this earth, my husband and I had the final responsibility of taking care of arrangements for her memorial. Exhausted and sad, we went to meet with the funeral home directors. When we sat down with the staff, we were informed that someone had paid for the cost of her memorial service. We couldn't believe it! Our minds were blown, and we both cried tears of happy gratitude. It was another undeserved, unexpected, and very much appreciated reminder of God's presence in our lives and in our pain. This debt that we owed, someone else paid on our behalf, out of nothing but love for us. Remember John 3:16? Jesus did that same thing—except he gave his actual life. For me and you. This was one of many ways—using the amazing angels around us—that God showed his love for me and my family.

After that season, I had a whole new love and appreciation for God. I felt how much he loved me and my family. It became so real, no longer an abstract idea I read about, but something I had lived and experienced. I felt closer to him after he carried me through that time, and I knew it was him who carried me because for the first time in my life I let him. Daily I talked to him, cried to him, and he showed his goodness over and over.

As awesome as that was, the story doesn't end there. Remember my troubled marriage? Well, after things settled down following my mother-in-law's passing, things got sorted out for my husband and me as well. Our relationship began to improve, and though I didn't know why, I was so glad! Then one day, at a family event, God put all the pieces together. A relative of my husband's got me alone for a minute and shared with me how he knew what we had been through had been hard for me, something I had never discussed with anyone. He knew this because years prior he and his wife had gone through something similar with his father. He said that during that time his wife showed so much love to her father-in-law that he was still to this day so grateful to her. He knew that, even though she loved her father-in-law, everything she did during that time was out of love for him, her husband.

At that moment, I realized God had used this tragic and grueling experience to heal my marriage. The discord in my marriage was due to many factors, not the least of which was that my husband had become convinced I no longer loved him. When my attention was called to the fact that my labor of love in caring for his mother was what God had used to mend our relationship, I was awestruck. Remember, I thought adding the care of a dying mother-in-law to our already stressful lives was the last thing we needed. When we are at our worst or weakest, we don't feel capable of taking on new or hard things, but the truth is we are never capable without God. It's only in his strength that we can do any of the things we do, because he is able. God took a time in my life when I had no strength left, and he became my strength. Not only that, he did "exceedingly abundantly" more.

Think about what we want for our loved ones or for our children. We don't want them merely to survive this crazy, cruel world; we want them to thrive. John 10:10 tells us Jesus came not so that we can merely survive but so that we can have abundant lives! God didn't just want me to survive this season and move on; he fully intended to use it to heal me and help me experience life abundantly. What I thought would surely kill me, God used to *heal* me.

It was this lived experience, and the realization of God's mighty hard and loving presence in every single gut-wrenching moment, that made me fall head over heels in love with him. It's what took me from the girl who was seeking to know God's love and acceptance to the woman who is so in love with God that she'll gladly do anything he asks. Whereas I once struggled to submit (and unfortunately sometimes still do), I now know that anything a loving God asks of me is for my good. Witnessing God's love poured out on me and my family made me *want* to love him back, more than any other selfish desire I might have. Since that time, my motivation to do all the things I do has been different.

So, what does all this falling in love have to do with wellness? Our heart is the driving force behind everything our body does. Many other organs and parts do important things, but the heart is what supplies nutrients to every one of those organs. With every beat of our heart, blood is circulated to the rest of our body. If the heart stops beating for a few seconds, we won't survive. If our heart even slows down too much, we will be weakened and unable to do what we need and want to do.

In the same way, our figurative heart is the driving force behind our physical, mental, spiritual, and emotional wellness. If our heart is fixed on God and we're head over heels in love with him, then our heart will be beating at the perfect tempo to help us thrive. What does the Bible say about our heart?

- "Guard your heart above all else, for it is the source of life" (Proverbs 4:23 CSB). Our heart is a life source, the root of our motivation, and it needs to be protected.

- "A person's heart plans his way, but the Lord determines his steps" (Proverbs 16:9 CSB). God has already laid a path for us and enabled us to walk it, and what we set our heart on will determine which route we take and our motivation to start walking.
- "A joyful heart is good medicine, but a broken spirit dries up the bones" (Proverbs 17:22 CSB). A heart filled with the joy of the Lord contains healing power, but allowing our spirit to be broken takes the life-giving marrow from our bones. In other words, having the joy of the Lord helps us be motivated to be well, even when we are hurting.
- "Take delight in the Lord, and he will give you your heart's desires" (Psalm 37:4 CSB). A heart that loves the Lord so much that it delights in him will see its desires fulfilled (and one that loves the things of this world will not).

The reason we needed to start a book on wellness with a discussion of falling in love with Jesus is because there is no more powerful motivator than unconditional, head-over-heels, crazy love. Our society's track record of failed resolutions each year prove our motivation can be lacking, and uncovering better motivation for wellness is a first step in the right direction.

What does *my* story of falling in love have to do with *your* motivation to be well and make good choices? Remember Maslow and his theory? He said that humans' first motivation is to meet the most basic needs, and only when those needs are met can we be motivated to do the things that truly fulfill us. Ironically, if we are constantly trying to survive, and never getting to the part where we are doing the things that we were made to do, we will always feel unfulfilled. That's where Jesus comes in. What Maslow didn't account for, God did. God is the perfect provider, the most loving companion and friend, and he is more than able to "exceedingly abundantly" meet our every need. If we are women who are in love with Jesus, then we trust that he is with us and for us, and will do what he promises.

The problem is, we are not perfect, and our humanity likes to rear its ugly face in the name of survival and self-preservation when times get tough. My typical response to anything that threatens my safety, or that of my family, is a combination of paralyzing rumination and extreme strategizing. Neither of those are necessary or helpful, and both are detrimental to the pursuit of wellness. In fact, Paul tells us, "Don't worry about anything, but in everything, through prayer and petition with thanksgiving, present your requests to God. And the peace of God, which surpasses all understanding, will guard your hearts and minds in Christ Jesus" (Philippians 4:6–7 CSB).

Therein lies the secret to bypassing our motivation to take care of the basics first. God's already got it. He even tells us to let him handle it, and if we do, we will no longer worry but be at peace, despite anything we are lacking at the moment. This heart-guarding peace, which comes from a complete devotion to and reliance on the God we love, is what frees us to *want* to make the best choices. Life certainly requires our time and attention to basic needs. We have to pay the bills, cook dinner, and do the things that make up daily life. Our family's difficult season of life when my mother-in-law was dying still required a constant fulfillment of daily obligations to those around me. This verse doesn't give us a pass to sail on by our responsibilities; it gives us freedom not to worry if we have a need that is not yet met. It lets us know we have access to the kind of peace that will protect our hearts and minds from the wear and tear that life's worries can bring. This assurance of God's presence in and power over everything from our daily bread to our biggest accomplishments squashes our human need for self-preservation before self-actualization. We are driven by love, not controlled by fear. This love of God and the peace he provides frees us to pursue being our best selves and living our best lives, even when we are not (yet) sure how today's needs are going to be met.

I don't know what your story is. Perhaps you aren't sure God has ever shown up for you like he did for me. Maybe you know you aren't truly in love with Jesus, but you're thinking about it for the first time. Praise Jesus for divine curiosity! Keep going on this journey with me and God, and I'm confident your heart will be impacted. Maybe you've had a similar experience where you endured a time when God showed you who he is and how much he loves you. I'm so happy to share in your joy and gratitude. Maybe you experienced hardships, but you are still angry with God because you feel like he didn't show up on your behalf. Sweet sister, if that is the case, my heart hurts for you and you are not alone. I urge you to read the verses above and see the love God has embedded in them. God loves you, and he is waiting for you to pour out the things you've been clinging to into his divine care. That's not an easy process, but it is abundantly beneficial, and there is help in later chapters especially for you.

<hr>

We are made to love God with everything we are. It's a daily choice, and it's something that has grown in me more and more as I've drawn nearer to him. This love and the want-to that comes with it are things I cannot give you. If you've got it, I'm so happy for you! If you're not sure you've fallen in love with God, please know: you will receive no judgment from me. I've been there. God doesn't need us pretending we feel what we don't. If you'll take what love you do have and pray that God would increase it, seeking him earnestly, he will. I promise, he is simply waiting for you to ask!

Whatever love for God you've got, let *that* be your motivation to keep reading this book. The desire to be a certain size, achieve a particular goal, or overcome a bad habit can be motivating for a time. Eventually, it will fade. Only a heart that is truly in love with Jesus will be motivated to seek wellness in all circumstances.

Reflection
1. Think back to any previous attempts you have made to better your health. What was your motivation?
2. How would you describe your feelings for Jesus?
3. What step can you take today, from wherever you are right now, to grow your love for Jesus? (Examples: start your day with gratitude, listen to worship music each morning, ask God daily to help you see his presence in your life, etc.)

THE WELL WOMAN

3 SANCTIFIED GROUND

They say Rome wasn't built in a day, and I've heard many friends proclaim they are a work in progress. Anyone who lives in or has traveled through central Texas will tell you that I-35 is always and forever a work in progress. It takes time and consistent effort to build something great like the city of Rome, and all that time and effort resulted in a city that benefited her people and left a legacy that is still there today. Until we get to heaven, we are all works in progress. Think of the women in your life. That woman you admire who seems to have it all together, the friend who can't seem to stop self-sabotaging, and every woman in between have one thing in common: they are works in progress. We all are.

Our culture is all about progression, becoming better at what we do and who we are and working toward the next best thing. Bigger, better, and more are what we are encouraged to seek. The work in progress I'm referring to, the thing God's Word beckons us to, is something different. Progress has nothing to do with fame, fortune, or the next big thing, and everything to do with doing the next right thing to become more like Jesus. Romans 5:1 says we are justified through faith, meaning God has pardoned us—in other words, he has offered us a pass on the punishment we deserve. All we have to do is profess our faith in Jesus. That first step of acceptance and believing that Christ died for us justifies us, makes us right with him. There is nothing we can do to be more saved— and certainly nothing we can do to lose our salvation. It is a done deal. In John 17, Jesus was preparing to die for us, in order to save us so we could have this justification. Jesus actually prayed to God on our behalf and asked him to sanctify us as well. Being sanctified means becoming holy. Jesus wanted us to become more like him, and he knew it would be a process, one he was willing to pay a high price to ignite. "I sanctify myself for them, so that they also may be sanctified by the truth" (John 17:19 CSB).

We are *justified* by faith in Christ, and we are *sanctified* by the Word of God and knowing what is true about him. So, this process and our progress in this life are all meant to make us more and more holy, preparing us for the day that we will be with God in heaven and become truly holy. The thought of it sends shivers up my spine! God put in place a plan that would take this hot mess of a woman and not only save me but make me closer and closer to being holy! And though I may make mistakes along the way, one day I will become holy, I will sit in his actual presence and be *truly* holy. That's so exciting and beats the heck out of any fancy house or earthly fame I could ever lust after.

All right then. We've been justified, and we are being sanctified, but how does this progressive sanctification work? I'm so glad you asked, and I'm even more glad God has provided an answer to that very question.

Psalm 92:13 tells us to be planted in the Lord so we can flourish. Better yet, Psalm 1:1–3 says that those who are planted by water will be blessed, will bear fruit in their season, and will not wither. I want to flourish, bear fruit, and be able to stand the tests that certain seasons bring. But how? That's the question this chapter sets out to answer.

How can we establish sanctified ground upon which we can become a well woman?

We've already discussed that becoming well starts with our own personal motivation, and the best way to become well is to be motivated by our love for Jesus. Part of loving God is getting to know him. The more we know of God, the more of his character we come to understand, and the more like him we can become. I like the analogy of a tree that is planted by water. Trees have roots that need water and nutrients in order to survive and continual access to these things to flourish. When a tree is planted, it takes time, years even, for its roots to establish well enough to provide support for its lifetime. The God who made trees knows exactly how they work, and he's the same God who made us and gave us the Psalms above as an example to follow. We, like the tree, need to plant ourselves on solid ground where we will be nourished and able not only to survive but to *flourish*. That is what a well woman does.

In order for us to be planted, rooted, and able to grow in sanctification, I think there are three basic biblical truths we need to pack our soil with. Once we understand each one, we can work them into our solid and sanctified ground, building upon that ground in the chapters to come.

Truth #1: Identity

Who are you? That is the question identity asks, and it's a monumental inquiry. Having a clear answer is a prerequisite to flourishing. It is so easy to fall into a pattern of mistaken identity. Sometimes the world tries to tell us who we are. When we listen, problems arise. The world told me I was smart, so if I ever did anything stupid, I felt like a fraud and a hypocrite, like I had lost my identity. The world also told me, in not so direct terms, that there are some things I can't do because I am a woman. I believed the world and saw myself as being limited to certain roles, and incapable of moving beyond them. Fortunately, I've had some benevolent and empowering friends and mentors who have identified talents in me and helped me to see and use them.

If I'm being honest, I don't need the world to help me misidentify who I am, as I do a fantastic job all by myself. I have found my identity wrapped up in roles I've held, like being a mom or wife. I've allowed jobs to define who I am, and my successes or failures to determine how well I'm living my identity. Every time God calls me to end a chapter or a season by leaving a job or volunteer role that I have loved and poured into, I have to allow him to remind me that my identity is not in that role, that I am still who he says I am no matter how or where he chooses to use me.

If mistaken identity creates distraction and barriers for us, and knowing who we are is required to be a well woman, we'd better figure out how to put away our false impressions and identify who we truly are.

"Acknowledge that the Lord is God. He made us, and we are his—his people, the sheep of his pasture" (Psalm 100:3 CSB).

God says we are his, made to follow him like sheep follow a shepherd. We trust he will lead us to the right place, provide for us, guide us, and pursue us when we are lost. When sheep know they belong to the shepherd, they look for him always.

"I have been crucified with Christ, and I no longer live, but Christ lives in me. The life I now live in the body, I live by faith in the Son of God, who loved me and gave himself for me" (Galatians 2:20 CSB).

Christ lives in us, and we live by faith in him. We are not only his followers; we are his vessels, allowing the love he fills us with to pour out onto everything we do.

"Now you are the body of Christ, and individual members of it" (1 Corinthians 12:27 CSB).

Paul, one of the most prominent early Christian teachers, tells us that as Christ followers we collectively make up the body of Christ, and each of us is an individual member. That means we are not in competition but are a coordinated effort serving the same God and on the same mission. We each have a role, and we are all in this together.

We are his, he is in us, and we are all part of a greater plan to represent Jesus to the world. We are daughters of the King. That is who we are, and we have to plant that seed of truth firmly in our sanctification soil and water it regularly. Everything we do has to align with this identity, and if it doesn't, then we shouldn't do it. A well woman knows who she is and lives accordingly.

Truth #2: Worthy

That little word has significant implications. Most of us are willing to give generously our time, money, and talents for worthy causes. In this busy life where opportunities and needs abound, we have to decide which causes are worthy enough to get our attention. Merriam-Webster defines worth as "the value of something measured by its qualities or by the esteem in which it is held." Worth is something every woman wants.

Worthiness in our world is often determined by success, accomplishments, and affluence. I read a story once about a pastor who dressed as a homeless person and camped outside his own church while recording the experience on video. Time and time again, churchgoers walked right by him. Why? They didn't deem him worthy. Lack of worth is something we fear, because we know in our own humanity, we are offenders at assigning greater worth to certain people over others.

Sometimes we determine worthiness by good deeds. People are esteemed and noticed because they do something selfless, heroic, or altruistic. This is wonderful, but unfortunately it can sometimes lead us to feel unworthy because we have not done anything that we determine to be at the level of the deeds of the esteemed. For this reason I felt so completely unworthy of God's love that I avoided seeking it for a long time.

What does God say about how worthy we are of his love and affection?

"But God proves his own love for us in that while we were still sinners, Christ died for us" (Romans 5:8 CSB).

God says we are worthy of his love. Despite our imperfections, we are so worthy in his eyes that he gave his son to die for us.

"But he said to me, 'My grace is sufficient for you, for my power is perfected in weakness'" (2 Corinthians 12:9 CSB).

Our weakness is not an indication of a lack of worth; it's an opportunity for God's power to be perfected. He has deemed us worthy, a perfect match for his strength, and he wants to work through us to impact his kingdom.

God isn't like us; he doesn't deem certain people more worthy than others. His Word tells us he sees our imperfections and he loves us all. No deed can earn or undo his love. I want you to read the following sentence as many times as you need to until you believe it.

I am worthy of God's love.

Truth #3: Valuable

We know now that we are worthy of God's love, but how worthy are we? This is the question of value. Have you ever felt unseen? Does it ever seem like everyone around you is getting what they need and want aplenty, and you are the only one suffering?

Genesis 16 tells us about a woman who likely felt like that. Hagar was a slave to Sarai (later named Sarah). When God had yet to deliver on his promise to Sarai and Abraham to give them a child, Sarai had a plan to speed things up. She decided Abraham should sleep with Hagar to get her pregnant, and as Sarai's slave, the child would then inherently belong to Sarai and Abraham. Obviously, this plan was all kinds of flawed, but what I want us to see right now is Hagar. The story goes on to say that once Hagar did become pregnant, Sarai began to mistreat her so badly that she ran away. Alone, used, abused, and powerless, I can imagine that Hagar felt anything but valuable. She certainly was not valuable to those around her.

It was at this point, when she was isolated in the wilderness, that God presented himself to her, telling her of his great plans for her and her son. She said, "In this place, have I actually seen the one who sees me?" (Genesis 16:13 CSB). There it is, what she was wanting. She does mean something to someone, to the one who sees her. She is so valuable to him that he chased her down and made sure she knew that she was seen, known, and important. Later, Hagar again finds herself alone, after Sarah sent her away. This time Hagar's baby had grown into a young boy. After some time, they had run out of food and water, and she was now in the wilderness, convinced she was alone and that her son was going to die. God appeared to her again and rescued her. God saw her, she was valuable to him, just as valuable as Abraham and Sarah. You are also valuable to God, as valuable as any other woman, even those who seem more favored than you at the moment.

How valuable does God say you are?

"Aren't five sparrows sold for two pennies? Yet none of them is forgotten in God's sight. Indeed, the hairs of your head are all counted. Don't be afraid; you are worth more than many sparrows" (Luke 12:6–7 CSB).

You are more valuable to God than any creature. Like the sparrow, the world may make you feel common or invaluable, but God never will. You are so precious to him that he has taken the time to count every hair on your head. You, my friend, are valuable beyond measure.

A well woman knows her identity is in Christ, knows she is worthy of being loved, and believes she is valuable to God. These truths are what she uses to fertilize her soil. She draws from them repeatedly, as an endless supply of strength that sustains her. They enable her to grow in this sanctification process, day after day and year after year.

Reflection
1. Think about how you identify yourself. After reading about your identity in Christ, write a description of your identity.

2. Sometimes we become convinced of false identities, or that we are not worthy of love, or not valuable. After reading this chapter, write one lie you have believed about yourself.

3. Pray over the lie you just wrote. Write down how you think God would respond to that lie. What would he say to you about it?

4 WATER AND SUNLIGHT

So far on our wellness journey we have established a strong foundational love for the Lord and a knowledge of what his Word says to be true of us. I believe these things alone are enough to empower us to start making changes that will help us in becoming well women. What's next is to figure out how to take what we've established and use it as fuel and guidance on this journey. A well woman doesn't simply know who she is and how precious she is to her Creator. She takes what she knows to be true and lives by these things. If we are to be truly well, we have to . . .

1.   know what God says,
2.   believe what God says,
3.   and live by what God says.

If we are to do those three things, we need to hear God. He is our guide, our shepherd. How do we hear God? So many women before us have asked that question, and I'm proposing two simple actions: seeking and listening.

Let's start with seeking. We seek God to know, have a relationship with, and hear him. Compellingly, the more we seek, the more we will know him; the better we know him, the closer our relationship with him becomes; and the more we nurture our relationship with him, the better able to hear him we will be. Think about it this way: what if a stranger jumped out in front of a car in order to save your life. You would be grateful; you might even want to get to know this person, get their phone number, or friend request them on social media. Then, let's say life went on and you were busy (I know it's hard to imagine that life would get hectic, but go with me here). Let's say you didn't talk to this person for a while, until around the holidays when you thought you should reach out and wish them a merry Christmas. Maybe you occasionally like their social media posts, reminisce with a friend about the day they saved your life, but beyond that you don't involve this person in your day-to-day living. I think we can both agree that what I have described is not a meaningful relationship. You have no idea what this person likes, what their qualities are, how they take their eggs, or what their dislikes are. In order to have an actual relationship, you would have to invest some time and attention and make an effort to get to know them. That's what we need to do with God, and this is where seeking him comes in as a way to continue to feed our roots and grow.

How do we go about seeking God? I've found four key ways to do this, and they require nothing more than a willing heart to start doing on the regular, today!

First, pray.

The Bible tells us in so many passages to pray. Jesus prayed throughout his time on this earth, and one of the staples of any church service is prayer. Why? This is how we talk to God, connect with him, and how we invite him to speak to us. I encourage you to make prayer a part of your daily routine, and if you are already doing that, try working on improving the frequency, quality, or intimacy of your prayer time. Matthew 6:5–14 even gives us instructions on how to pray. God wants time alone with us, and we don't even have to know what to say because he already knows what we need. The Lord's Prayer is an example of how we should pray; God is so good that he gives us specific instructions to help us out (Matthew 6:9–13). This prayer example starts with acknowledging who God is, goes on to ask for provision and forgiveness, reminds us that we are also called to forgive others, and ends with a plea for protection from temptation and the devil himself. Finding God starts with prayer and flourishing requires regular doses of him. Think about your daily routine, and consider whether prayer is a pivotal part of every day. What could you do to improve or change your prayer life?

Second, read the Word.

"Take the helmet of salvation and the sword of the Spirit—which is the word of God," Ephesians 6:17 CSB). God's Word is more than a message to his people; it's more than a chronicle of the history of Christianity. It's the sword of the Spirit, a powerful weapon to pierce souls and defend our faith. Getting into the Bible is the only way we can learn to use this weapon effectively.

If you feel intimidated by reading the Bible on your own, you are not alone. The Bible is full of mysterious metaphors, parables, and references to things that, while still applicable today, are foreign concepts. So, what's a girl to do if she wants to be a sword-wielding well woman but doesn't know how? There are entire books written on this topic alone, but I'm certain I can offer you some help and encouragement in this short, simple segment. There are four effective strategies I've learned that are sure to increase your confidence in reading God's Word.

First, start with prayer. Invite the Lord to speak to you, guide you, and open your eyes, heart, and mind. He will never refuse an invitation by his beloved daughter (that's you, by the way). Second, read regularly. Remember the first time you put on makeup or walked in high heels? What about the first time you attempted to make a recipe from scratch? Or tried a new exercise? Most likely you would say these initial attempts were awkward at best and disastrous at worst. But with every subsequent attempt at each of the above, things became less awkward and more familiar, didn't they? The same is true of reading the Word: the more you read, the easier and better it gets! Third, don't try to eat the whole elephant at once. I don't know about you, but I like to eat my elephants bite by bite and a little each day. It takes years and years to eat a whole elephant that way, you might not even finish the entire elephant in a lifetime, but at least you have tasted each part, savored each bite, and allowed each bit to nourish you a little at a time. So, each day, pick a verse, a small passage, or a manageable section of a study. Do what you can. Be the tortoise, not the hare. Little by little, you will see progress.

Finally, get help. There are daily devotionals, Bible-based journals, and so many studies that can be your guide through the Bible. You can join a group and do a study with others, start a group, ask a more seasoned Christian friend to help you, follow an online blog—the options for help are endless. Just make sure you know that the Bible is the original source of truth, and anything else you read or study should align with God's Word and enhance your understanding. Avoid anything that contradicts or challenges the Word, inviting Satan's interference.

Prayer and reading God's Word are the first two ways we can strengthen our roots and grow in this sanctification process. The third way to seek God is to do it continuously.

"Rejoice always, pray constantly, give thanks in everything; for this is God's will for you in Christ Jesus" (1 Thessalonians 5:16–18 CSB). The words of Paul are clear—words like *always, constantly,* and *in everything.* It's so easy to pray in the morning and forget all about that time with the Lord five minutes after we walk out the front door. Rejoicing and giving thanks in happy times comes easier than in hard times. Why would continuity be so important? Well, the opposite of continuous is intermittent, periodic, or sporadic. If we are trying to seek God to know him and become the well women he intends us to be, a periodic effort simply won't be as effective as a consistent one. Practically speaking, we can do this in many ways. Set a reminder on your phone to stop and pray, listen to Christian radio and podcasts while you are driving or working, or find a friend to encourage you to be more consistent. Think of one thing you can do differently that would help you be more consistent in seeking God.

The final key way to seek God is to find community.

"Two are better than one because they have a good reward for their efforts. For if either falls, his companion can lift him up. Also, if two lie down together, they can keep warm; but how can one person alone keep warm? And if someone overpowers one person, two can resist him. A cord of three strands is not easily broken" (Ecclesiastes 4:9–12 CSB). The author of this passage, thought to be David's son, King Solomon, gives a pretty convincing argument for community. We can accomplish more together, help each other when one gets down, and comfort each other when times get tough. Together, we can also unite to resist those who seek to overtake us. I don't know about you, but I want that kind of community!

Maybe you've already found your tribe, so you can check this one off. For those who are still looking, I want to encourage you. Even if you feel like a square peg trying to fit in a round hole, keep looking. God did not intend for you to be the only one going it alone. I am so sure of that, I'm willing to put it in writing. I've been there. Overlooked more often than noticed, betrayed by the few I let get close, and dismissed by the cool club for reasons I still don't know. Sound familiar? Keep seeking God continuously, and trust him to show you to your community. Invest in others and allow them to invest in you. Satan wants you isolated because he knows you are more vulnerable that way, and he plays on your insecurities and fears to keep you from the community that is ready and willing to empower you to be a well woman! Don't let him keep you from your tribe. Consider starting today by joining a new group, reaching out to a neighbor or friend, or joining a church if you don't already attend one.

A well woman is given the opportunity for growth and sanctification by hearing God. She does this by first seeking God in prayer, reading the Word, continuously pursuing these things, and being in community. Problem solved, time to move on, right? Not so fast.

A big part of my job is to diagnose. That's a fancy word for figuring out what is going on with someone, what the problem or issue is. One of the key ways I do this is by asking questions. These questions tell me more about the background of the problem and give important details that I wouldn't necessarily glean without asking. The crucial, most significant part of this process is not the questions or the process of elimination I go through to determine the correct diagnosis. Nope. The essential element of diagnosing and treating any condition is my ability to *listen*. It is in listening that I learn the critical information. It's in listening that I can hear the mention of otherwise unspoken and unsolicited details. It's in listening that I can hear the priorities of the individual that supersede any book knowledge or physiologic process. Without listening, asking questions is simply an interrogation, a one-sided inquisition. When we listen, we take pause to know what we did not know previously and to hear what we haven't anticipated. There is a huge difference between seeking and listening, and if we are to know, believe, and live by God's Word, we are going to have to learn to listen.

I am not a good listener by nature. My mind is always going in a million different directions, and my nature is to want to help. A desire to help is not a bad thing, unless the person simply wants to be heard rather than helped. I have had to learn to listen to the Lord and others, and I'll gladly share the methods I've acquired to do this.

I've learned to take pause. When in conversation with anyone or in prayer with the Lord, before speaking, I pause. This indicates to the other party that I'm listening and invites them to speak. A pause also reminds me to listen and not to focus on processing information and formulating a response. Pause is a powerful, deliberate call to two-way conversation, and it is a huge help when trying to hear God.

The Bible tells us, "Stop fighting, and know that I am God, exalted among the nations, exalted on the earth" (Psalm 46:10 CSB). Some translations say "Be still and know," but I think this version effectively brings the point home. Stop fighting, let go of being right, forget about being heard, get over winning, and know that he is God and we are not. Taking pause and letting go of the fight makes us open and ready for an encounter with the Lord, just like pausing to listen helps me understand my patients. There are times that I've encountered God in the most surprising ways, but if I'm seeking him, then I should do everything in my power to be ready for an encounter. In fact, I need to anticipate hearing God and have faith that he is going to speak to me. I find it helpful to ask God to help me in this, to give me ears to hear and a heart ready to receive what he has to say.

If hearing God was as easy as seeking and actively listening, we would all be getting divine words all day long, and we would never have any reason to struggle with living by God's Word. Unfortunately, there is one final issue to address in this mission to hearing God: ignoring the noise.

What is this noise? Oh, I think you know. Noise is anything that makes it hard for us to hear God. Sometimes noise is distraction, like social media or the opinions of others. The story of Mary and Martha comes to mind (Luke 10:38–42). Jesus had come to visit, and Martha wanted everything to be perfect. She was cooking the food and setting the table, doing all the things, while her sister Mary was sitting at Jesus's feet. When Martha got tired of doing it all herself and asked Jesus to get Mary to help her, Jesus lovingly let her know she was focusing on the wrong thing. She let the business of serving distract her from the presence of the Lord. I don't know about you, but when my to-do list is calling my name, it is a constant effort not to let it be louder than God, but I assure you it is possible. We have already talked about taking pause to listen to God. If you are feeling overworked and stressed about all the things on your list, that is a definite call to pause at the feet of Jesus.

Sometimes the things that distract us are things we put before God, which the Bible refers to as idols. Luke 6:24 says "woe to you who are rich, for you have received your comfort" (CSB). If we allow the comforts of this world to be more important than God, we will surely have a hard time hearing him. I've let my ego drown out the voice of God, allowed the desire for material things to outweigh my desire for the Lord, and fueled my need for security by seeking money over God. All of these are examples of idols, and they dampen our ability to hear God.

Trials in life can also be a distraction from hearing the Lord, if we let them. My instinct in a trial is to fight, take action, and take control of the situation. Talk about distraction! If I'm trying to handle things (like Martha), then I am going to have a hard time being still and listening to the Lord.

"Be sober-minded, be alert. Your adversary the devil is prowling around like a roaring lion, looking for anyone he can devour" (1 Peter 5:8 CSB). One of the craftiest distractions is Satan himself. He convinced Eve she was missing out when she famously ate that apple, telling her that God was holding out on her, keeping her from something good (Genesis 3:4–6). Fear of Missing Out, or FOMO as it's commonly referred to these days, is alive and well; they even make FOMO T-shirts! Satan distracted Eve by telling her God had misled her or lied to her (Genesis 3:1, 4–5). I've let Satan convince me that what God tells me not to do really isn't that bad for me. I've even let him convince me that what the world has for me is better than what God has. Satan is still up to his old tricks, isn't he? How has he been able to distract you? The more we are aware of his tricks, the more quickly we can put on our God-given noise-canceling headphones and hear the voice of truth that lives in us!

All of the types of noise we've discussed so far are from external sources. What about the noise that comes from within us? Self-doubt, fear, self-criticism, and lack of faith in God are a few of the internal noises I've faced. Have you ever felt the call to do something but allowed fear, doubt, anxiety, or lack of faith to stop you? We've all been there, and unfortunately we can be our own worst enemy at times.

Before we become discouraged about all this, let's remind ourselves of what we are talking about: noise. That's all it is, just noise. Noise has no power to change our behavior in and of itself. Satan doesn't either, by the way. So, how do you deal with noise? It starts with what we've already discussed—seeking and listening. The more we do that, the better we hear God, and the less we hear the noise. Sometimes it gets tricky and we wonder if what we are hearing is noise or from the Lord, so how do we discern? Romans 12:2 says that if we allow God to renew our minds, we will be able to discern his will. Prayer is powerful and effective, and asking God to renew us each day helps us in discerning.

We can also look for confirmation that we are following the will of God. This often comes in the form of open doors, sometimes even with little to no effort on your part. When I was pregnant with my first child, I once had a craving for a candy bar. I was at home, no candy bar in sight, and sitting on my couch wishing I had one. Then I heard a knock at the door, and when I opened it a little girl stood outside holding one of those glorious boxes of chocolate bars that kids sell. It was divine, and I bought two! That is the kind of confirmation I am talking about: something happens that you cannot explain, and it is exactly what your heart desires or just what you need to take the next step.

Other ways I find confirmation are multiple sources telling me the same thing, which matches what I already feel almost certain I'm hearing from the Lord. For example, in a time of transition or change, I will pray over the options or different paths. Sometimes in my time of prayer I feel a pull toward one direction or option, but other times I don't. Inevitably, when I open my Bible, there will be something in the passage that speaks to my situation, and I get a clue. Then I'll hear a song on the radio on the way to work that reinforces what I've read. Sometimes I'll even have a random stranger or a coworker who has no idea what I'm struggling with who says something applicable to the situation. Individually these clues don't mean a lot, but when they align with what I feel the Lord is already telling me, they become a noise-cancelling confirmation.

The final way I've experienced divine confirmation of God's will is peace. I am a planner, and I like to have steps laid out so I can anticipate and be prepared. God doesn't always work like that; in fact, he usually calls us to step out in faith, trusting that he has it all planned out. When I am walking in the will of God, I have a sense of peace, even in the midst of situations that would normally cause me great anxiety.

So, once you have sought God and spent some time trying to listen to him, look for confirmation in the form of open doors, outside sources reinforcing the same thing you feel the Lord telling you, and peace that you have no business feeling in this situation, yet you do.

In this process of noise-cancelling confirmation, don't forget to heed the warning in 1 Peter 5:8. Satan will surely be there with his noisy self. Barriers that come up are not always an indication that you are on the wrong track. If you come across something in your way, stop and pray. God will remove it or give you a way around it if you are meant to keep going.

I was recently involved in a major transition in my church, and I was very excited about it. The church was in the process of transitioning from being a satellite church under the umbrella of a parent church to being an independent church. During this time I ran across several people who questioned the details of this transition, and I didn't necessarily have answers for their questions. There was even one encounter where I felt personally attacked by a woman at an event where I was representing our church. These experiences caused me to question whether I was on the right track. I quickly started to pray about this, and it wasn't long before I realized this was an attack by Satan, not a God-given call to change direction.

There are times I feel particularly under attack, where repeated setbacks and struggles start to get me down, despite repeated prayer and seeking God. These times call for powerful noise-cancelling techniques. When the noise starts to get to me, I have learned to proclaim God's truths out loud and tell Satan he is not welcome. That's right, I say out loud things like "God is good" and "You are here in this place, Lord." Then I follow up these power statements with "Satan, get away, you slimy, powerless snake!" I urge you to try it for yourself. Speak what you know to be true and declare God's presence in your home, over your family, and in any situation. Works every time, not necessarily to change the situation, but it always sets me free from attack.

We absolutely have the power, through the Holy Spirit within us, to block out the noise.

The only way a well woman can live by what she knows is to seek the Lord and hear his voice louder than any other. Developing consistent habits around prayer, reading the Word, and seeking community are more than good Christian checklists to her. She works at weaving all of these into the continuous flow of her days, weeks, months, and years. These are the methods she uses to guide her steps and help her live out the love she has for Jesus. Her methods are not her own, and she has no privileged access to them that others are not also offered.

Seek God, hear him, and ignore the noise in your life today. These things are not easy, but they are requirements for being well, and you are most definitely able to do them, because he says so.

Reflection
1. Consider how you typically seek the Lord. What methods do you use and how often?
2. How could you improve the way you seek the Lord? Are you needing to increase the quantity or quality of time? List at least one thing you can start doing today to be better at seeking him.
3. We all have challenges with hearing the Lord; consider yours. Based on what you've read, what do you feel God calling you to do today to hear him better?

5 FORGIVEN AND FREED

As I have sought the Lord and learned to hear him, areas in my life and my heart in need of divine healing have been uncovered. I've found an example to illustrate the revelation and healing of hurt and sin: the hackberry tree. On a fairly regular basis I find a hackberry tree in my flower beds. If you are not familiar, hackberry trees are pesky weeds that grow in the form of trees; they are invasive and a nuisance. I enjoy taking good care of my expansive flower beds, and in spite of my best efforts, these things still show up. Now, in order to make things look nice, I may trim them down to where they are not visible to folks driving by, but if you look closely, the roots are still there. All it takes is a little rain, sun, and time, and soon they'll be back in full bloom again.

Hackberry trees are challenging to remove because their roots run deep and hold tight to the soil. Removal requires the laborious process of digging them out. What I have found most effective to eliminate the dreaded hackberry is to call John. John is our horticulture expert, and we usually have him come out once a year to trim everything and offer advice on how to manage our plants. I have to pay him extra to remove the hackberry trees, and it is worth every penny. I can't do it myself, especially because they are often embedded with other plants, plants I want to keep and not harm. Hopefully you are starting to see some parallels here. I call on John to rid me of my hackberry trees, and we call on Jesus to heal us in the areas of our life that have been invaded by unwanted things. That is exactly the point, yes, but there is so much more to this hackberry story.

Romans 3:23 says we have all sinned—in other words, we have all allowed our own hackberry trees to take root. John 16:20 promises we will have sorrow in this world, but those sorrows are only temporary compared to the eternal joy that awaits us in heaven. I find great hope in the biblical assurance that we all have hackberry trees, whether self-inflicted or not, and that God has plans to remove them permanently and bring us to a place where they don't exist. Philippians 1:29 points out that when we believe in Jesus and follow him, we will also suffer for him, and Psalm 34:19 reminds us even the most upstanding of Christians will face hardships, none of which are too big for God to handle. This little highlight reel just scratches the surface of how sufficiently God's Word acknowledges and addresses suffering.

Let's look at a biblical example of the hackberry tree metaphor and what Jesus did about it. "As he was teaching in one of the synagogues on the Sabbath, a woman was there who had been disabled by a spirit for over eighteen years. She was bent over and could not straighten up at all. When Jesus saw her, he called out to her, 'Woman, you are free of your disability.' Then he laid his hands on her, and instantly she was restored and began to glorify God" (Luke 13:10–13 CSB).

This story takes place in the synagogue as Jesus was teaching. We don't know if going to the synagogue was this unwell woman's regular practice or if perhaps she went there in hopes of being healed that day. She may have heard about Jesus's teachings and gone there to see him. Whatever the reason, it's worth noting she showed up where Jesus was. Her faith was not mentioned, and she didn't ask for healing, but Jesus knew what she needed. He called to her and initiated her healing on her behalf. Jesus knew her needs. It's important to consider what her condition was and what life was like for her because of it. Luke, the author telling her story, was a physician and reports her medical condition. Apparently, it was one that medicine could not heal. I can only imagine how being bent over would have interfered with everyday life. Talk about hackberry trees, this one was invasive and inhibiting. Basics like dressing and eating and bodily functions would have been difficult and likely painful. Social relationships must have been a challenge, as she could not look people in the eye. Did she have friends or family to help her? I hope so. What would it be like to never look up to the sky?

While I can't say I've experienced severe curvature of the spine, I can relate to a bent spirit and broken soul in need of a savior. Later in Luke 13, Jesus is talking to the leaders of the synagogue and compares what he has done for the woman to the untying of a donkey, freeing it to get water (Luke 13 15–16). Verse 16 says, "Satan has bound this woman" (CSB). The word *free* in "Woman, you are free of your disability" originated as a Greek word that means "to untie" (Luke 13:12 CSB). There is an emerging theme here of bondage versus freedom. Freedom comes through a God-given untying from that which binds us. Jesus healed this woman's soul first, by freeing her from being bound to Satan. We should take notice that what appears to be the issue in need of healing may not be what needs to be fixed first. Remember, there's no point in trimming the most visible part of a hackberry tree only to have the root remain. Once her soul was free, Jesus healed her body. The healing of our soul is often a prerequisite for physical healing.

Healing can take a long time (eighteen years for this woman). Sometimes, unlike this woman, we never get the full healing we want. We don't know that she was completely healed of all her pain and suffering, just that she was free of her disability and restored to glorify God. She may have continued to have pain related to her years of being stooped over or faced mockery from her community for her past. There are areas of suffering in my life that have yet to completely resolve, and likely this is true for most of us. Hebrews 12:7–11 says hardships can be discipline that God allows because he loves us. As a parent, I would love to upload all the wisdom I've gained in the school of hard knocks to my children so they do not have to suffer from making the same or similar mistakes as their mom. It doesn't work like that. Part of maturity is the process of enduring hardship. Romans 5:3–4 says suffering produces perseverance, which produces character, which produces hope. We can't forget that Christ himself suffered unjustly in order to give us hope. Sometimes there is suffering in this world that seems harsh and unjust. One of my daughter's friends was recently diagnosed with cancer. A twelve-year-old enduring chemotherapy and facing the big "C" seems cruel and unnecessary. I don't think anyone can tie up the reasoning behind suffering with a nice, neat bow. Some suffering is simply the reality of being in a fallen world, and a fulfillment of the warning provided to us in verses like Romans 3:23 and Psalm 34:19. What I am sure of is that Jesus sees our suffering and offers compassion and hope.

Of course, we have to mention the suffering we bring upon ourselves, also known as sin. Want to know something I learned about hackberry trees? The reason they seem to pop up out of nowhere is that their seeds get dropped on the ground, in the form of bird poop. Hackberry trees produce little berries that birds like to eat. Then, while perched on my other trees, the sweet little birdies do their business, dropping the remnants of those berries onto my soil. Before you know it, and most likely before it was even visible to the naked eye, that tiny seed sprouts into an invasive, unwanted, and unsightly weed. Sin is like that. The world, and our prowling tempter Satan, drop little harmless-appearing temptations in our lives that have the potential to grow if left unattended. Often it takes God to reveal the hidden things we are not even aware of. Once our sin is made known, it's up to us to act on that knowledge and remove the sin from our lives.

One of my spiritual struggles is this tug-of-war I like to do with God. It goes like this: I have a problem, and I try to solve it on my own for a bit; then I realize I need God's help. So I pray about it and ask God to help me, but even after I pray, I still to try to solve the problem on my own, as if God isn't capable of doing it and needs my help. I continue to have the same problem because I won't get out of the way and let God be God. I repeat this cycle wondering when God is going to help me until I realize he needs me to release my problems fully to him. The struggle will stop when I stop struggling to control things I was never meant to control. I finally humble myself, tell God I have realized the error of my ways (once again), and ask him to take this thing from me once and for all. Giving my problems to God is not an assurance of immediate resolution, though that can happen if it's God's will. Following my wholehearted release to God, problems may still exist, but I have a newfound peace about them.

Experiencing peace following release over and over has led me to understand that the root of my suffering isn't necessarily what it seems. I may not always have a choice in the things that come my way, but thankfully I have a choice in how I approach them. The root of my suffering isn't always the problem itself but my double-minded attempt to handle the problem on my own while claiming to have faith that God is the one in charge.

Our suffering is often rooted in and fertilized by sin. Although the problems we face may have nothing to do with our own choices, the sin in our hearts allows them to cause undue suffering.

Jesus is more powerful than Satan, and he already defeated sin on the cross. The stooped woman did not have the power to lift herself up, but Jesus does and he did. We are bent toward sin, and Jesus calls to us with intentions to lift us up to face him.

The first step to becoming free from our bondage is to turn to Jesus. Following the example of the woman in the synagogue, we have to acknowledge our hackberry trees. We must allow God to open our eyes to see them through whatever means necessary. Once they are acknowledged, we need to bring them to the feet of Jesus and leave them there. Words are not necessary; the woman in the synagogue didn't utter a single one. Simply the act of giving our pain, disabilities, wounds, challenges, frustrations, guilt, shame, and any other weighty burden to Jesus is all the invitation he needs. Resist the temptation to pick them back up or peel the label off to keep as a souvenir. Leave it all in his capable hands.

The purpose of releasing our sin to Jesus is for more than simply lightening our load. Jesus needs us to pour out ourselves to him and empty our hands because he's got a new load to give us. We now get to carry something so much better. It's called forgiveness. God knew we were going to sin, and he always had a plan to redeem us. He sent Jesus to die for us before we ever thought about repenting, while we were still living in our sin (Romans 5:8). Sin leads to death, and when we live a life driven by sin, we are dead, but God has given us life with Jesus and through Jesus (Ephesians 2:4–5). Forgiveness is the method God chose to deliver that life to us, and it's a badge of honor we get to wear humbly, a gift of mercy we don't deserve. Life is in him; death is in sin. Freedom, the same freedom that Jesus gave the woman in the synagogue, is available for us through forgiveness.

In Mark 2:1–12 there is a story of a paralyzed man whom Jesus healed.

"Seeing their faith, Jesus told the paralytic, 'Son, your sins are forgiven'" (Mark 2:5 CSB). This is another example of a time Jesus healed the soul before the body. Those who witnessed this questioned Jesus's authority to forgive sins, but in Mark 2:10 Jesus made it clear he absolutely had that authority. Jesus followed that proclamation up with more proof of who he was as he told the man to get up and walk, and immediately the man was able to do exactly that.

Even when we have been forgiven, we still own the freedom to choose our next steps. Sometimes I've chosen to go right back to that same cycle of sin. I've often done so out of shame, deciding that I'm too tarnished to do any good. But this line of thinking is so misguided, and it's a tool directly out of Satan's shed. God's Word tells us we are reconciled with God through Jesus's death, and once we have been forgiven, our sins are no longer counted against us (2 Corinthians 5:19). They are gone, erased. God no longer remembers them. We have to resist the temptation to go back and remember what God does not. Second Corinthians 5:17 says once we accept Christ as our savior, we are a new creation! The old me, the one who chose to live for worldly satisfaction and selfish desires, is dead. In Jesus I am new, shiny, and ready to walk a new way. It's time to move from a sin cycle to a win cycle, with Jesus. It takes daily choices to pick up that badge of forgiveness and seek him, and his mercies are new every single day. Forgiveness is offered to all of us; it's our choice to receive and walk in it.

God doesn't stop with forgiveness of sin; he offers healing as well. Many of us have wounds. We've already discussed the issue of sin, and though our sins are forgiven and erased, the wounds they can leave behind may need healing. Some wounds are not self-inflicted but created by this cruel world. Many of us have experienced trauma. According to the American Psychological Association, at least half of us will experience trauma at least once in our lives.[ii] Trauma comes from things like abuse or witnessing a violent act, and it can leave deep and painful wounds. Sometimes wounds come not from a painful infliction but more from a deprivation of nourishment. If we had unmet needs as a child, those become like a vitamin deficiency and can create lasting illness. Other needs for healing can arise from physical ailments, like those of the woman in Luke 13. As a health care provider, I see certain things on a daily basis. Everything from mild viruses to chronic and debilitating diseases cause suffering. Our specific types of healing needs may differ, but the overall need for healing is universal. That's the bad news. Thankfully, God offers good news regarding healing to all of us:

> The righteous cry out, and the Lord hears,
> and rescues them from all their troubles.
> The Lord is near the brokenhearted;
> he saves those crushed in spirit.

One who is righteous has many adversities,
but the Lord rescues him from them all. (Psalm 34:17–19 CSB)

As I've already mentioned, God has the power to heal anything, and sometimes he does, as in the case of the disabled woman in Luke 13 or the paralyzed man in Mark 2. Sometimes he doesn't offer complete healing of our condition, as is the case for anyone suffering from lifelong mental illness or chronic pain, for example. Eventually, we will all be healed in every way when he calls us home to be with him. Until then, especially in those cases where the condition persists, he offers healing in different forms. Psalm 34:17–19 above tells us God hears us, and don't we all want to be acknowledged and heard? I've learned that it's of utmost importance for my patients to know I have heard them. Though they would like a cure, they can accept the news that I don't have one if they know I understand and sympathize with their suffering. The passage goes on to say that not only does God hear us, but he also rescues us. Notice it doesn't say he changes our circumstances. He may not change the behavior of a demeaning boss, but he will rescue us from their effect on us, if we let him. God has yet to take away my tendency toward anxiety, but he anchors me with his Word and soothes me with his compassion when I am anxious. There is comfort in the presence of a loving heavenly Father, and he saves us when we are crushed in spirit. At times when I've endured loss that seemed too painful to bear, he has always shown up in one way or another. Make no mistake, there will be times when our spirit is crushed. It's those times when we feel backed into a corner or buried in a deep hole that we have no choice but to turn to him. We are crushed, but God makes all things new. It occurs to me that sometimes starting over is easier than replacing broken parts. If God allows us to be stripped of all worldly assurance, then we are left with complete reliance on him, and doesn't that benefit us more than a life void of suffering? Finally, the Psalms tell us that we will face adversity and lots of it. The passage doesn't say *some* or even *a moderate amount*. It says we will have *many* adversities. It also says that God, the one who loves us so much he sent his son to die for us, will rescue us from *every single one*.

While we don't always receive healing in the timing or form that we would like, we do all receive healing in the presence, comfort, rescue, and forgiveness of our Lord and Savior. Simply knowing this and saying it out loud brings a sense of freedom to my heart. If there is something you have been longing for God to fix and it has not happened, I challenge you to pray for God to free you from the bondage of the problem rather than heal the problem itself. Allow him to untie you, and get ready to walk in healing!

Let's go back to the woman in Luke 13. She was first freed from the bondage of her disability and then restored physically. The very next thing she did was to glorify God. What a beautiful example of accepting and walking in God's healing. I've also come up with a list of things she didn't do, which happens to be things I tend to do after a trial or season of suffering. Here they are, in no particular order:

- She didn't lament all the years she suffered.
- She didn't question God's methods.
- She didn't lecture God on his timing.
- She didn't conceal the fact from those around her that she had been suffering and subsequently healed.
- She didn't let anyone or anything convince her she was unworthy, too damaged, or not valuable enough for healing.
- She didn't go back to her old, sad, bent-over position.

This woman accepted the healing that was offered, when it was offered, and used it to bring glory to God. I see examples of this everywhere around me. There is a family in my town who started a nonprofit to help teens after their own teenage daughter committed suicide. I am sure they would give anything to have their beloved daughter back, and that is one of those hard losses none of us can explain. They are choosing to accept the healing God has offered them and walk in obedience to God, unbound by their loss and pain. One of the hardest things I do as an author is to share the most painful parts of my life with my readers. When I do share the things I would rather keep private, I always find the impact on readers is incredible, worth every bit of the courage it takes to put myself out there.

It is healing for others to see God's healing in you. Bringing him glory doesn't have to happen in public, though it might. You can bring him glory by praying with a friend, sending a text or card of encouragement to a friend enduring something you've already walked through, or by telling your story of healing to a coworker. Although I don't know God's call on your life to bring him glory, I can assure you it won't reach its full potential if you don't accept and walk in the healing God has given you.

A commitment to walking as a healed woman is the first of many steps on our journey to being well. God would never call us to do something he doesn't plan to equip us for, and bringing him glory by accepting and walking in our healing is no different than any other calling. God's Word tells us that he doesn't stop at forgiving and healing us; he also covers us. Jesus has our back, literally. Jesus came to bring sinners to repentance, not call those who are already sinless, or righteous (Luke 5:32). I have a tendency to think I'm not good enough to walk as forgiven and freed, because I remember all the wrong I've done, and sometimes I'm afraid others remember too. God says I am good enough, and he will show the world exactly what he has done with me to make it so.

As Isaiah says, "I rejoice greatly in the Lord, I exult in my God; for he has clothed me with garments of salvation and wrapped me in a robe of righteousness, as a groom wears a turban and as a bride adorns herself with her jewels" (Isaiah 61:10 CSB). Isaiah was a prophet who shares what it's like to be anointed by God's Spirit and called to bring good news to others (Isaiah 61:1). Being clothed with salvation and wrapped in righteousness is a pretty big deal, comparable to the coverings and accessories a bride and groom wear to prepare to join in marriage. The metaphor couldn't be more applicable. Without God we are all sinners living in this broken world and displaying our flaws when we behave badly. When we accept Jesus as our Savior, he comes into our hearts and gives us his Holy Spirit to dwell within us. This passage tells us there is more to the story. The heart that is committed to the Lord can also be made to appear godly on the outside. The person under those coverings isn't smothered or minimized, simply improved and transformed from the inside out, and in the process, takes on the appearance of salvation and righteousness. Do you see how important setting down those sins and burdens at the feet of Jesus is? In return we receive forgiveness, healing, and a covering of righteousness and salvation! Of course, we always have the option to go back and pick that nastiness back up and wear those old rags, but who wants to?!

Once the woman in the synagogue and the paralyzed man became spiritually and physically healed, they immediately impacted those around them. Luke 13:17 says the whole crowd was rejoicing because of what Jesus had done, and Mark 2:12 says the crowd was "astounded and gave glory to God" (CSB). I think it's important to know what joy can come from being free, for you and those around you. Sometimes when we are suffering and we look at the world around us, it seems everyone else is thriving. Your friend's Instagram-worthy photos that look so perfect are likely staged and not representative of reality. God's Word says there will be times the world seems to have joy when you don't. That type of joy is temporary and does not compare to the eternal joy we are promised with God forever. The knowledge that I am assured a place in heaven brings me joy, and the freedom that comes from God's untying of all that has bound me gives me a taste of that joy here on earth. When we allow ourselves to be ruled by the Holy Spirit we have received, we get to experience joy and pass it on to others (Galatians 5:22). In fact, when we walk with God on the path he calls us to, his mere presence with us brings "abundant joy" (Psalms 16:11 CSB).

If you think back to my description of a well woman, you might remember this line: she is beautiful to behold. That one brings me to tears because I have not always believed those words about myself and sometimes still struggle to do so today. I look in the mirror and see my flaws, and I look back in time and see all the ways I've messed up. But God does not. I don't know how you would describe yourself, and I want you to consider for a moment what words you would choose. How do you see yourself? Would beautiful be a word in your description? I can assure you, God thinks you are more than a sight for sore eyes; you are gorgeous to *his* eyes, a beauty to behold. He loved you so much he gave his son's life for you, to free you from your mistakes and wounds. He takes your heavy burdens and replaces them with forgiveness and joy. He even adorns you with his goodness so that others can see how beautiful you are. You, my friend, are beautiful to behold.

Romans 6:22 says that freedom from sin and becoming instead enslaved to God results in a process of becoming holy. The hackberry trees in my flower beds are completely removable, yet the challenges that we find rooted in our lives may not be. We are all works in progress, and certain areas may not find complete resolution in this lifetime, but a well woman knows she is not bound by her problem areas. Even wounds that heal leave scars, and the world may remember every terrible thing we have ever done. Yet being forgiven and freed is God's merciful enabling of a woman to be well despite the fact that she is flawed and scarred. It makes us all beautiful to behold.

Reflection

1. Write down something you have been longing for God to heal. If you don't have a specific prayer for yourself, write down a prayer of healing you've been long praying for someone else. Tell God your feelings about this particular hackberry tree; pour them all out to him.

2. Now ask God to free you or your loved one from the burden of the issue above rather than completely remove the issue itself. Ask him to reveal to you any barriers to freedom and ways you can allow him to lead you around them.

3. Sin is often defined as anything that comes between us and God. Is there a sin in your life you need to drop at the feet of Jesus? Seek God's clarity on this, and pray for him to reveal your sinful hackberry trees. Once you see them, leave them at the feet of Jesus, ask for forgiveness, and be ready to walk as a new creation.

38

6 LIVING ON PURPOSE

I'm thrilled, maybe even giddy, to walk you through taking hold of what we've covered thus far and carrying it into what's next. We've done some deep digging in the previous chapters, laid a strong foundation for becoming a well woman, and I want to take a moment to reflect on our wellness journey. So far, we have covered the following:

- We love God with everything we've got, or at least we're working on developing a relationship with him that will lead to an ever-increasing and all-consuming love.
- We now know our identity, worth, and value are in Christ.
- We know the steps to living out the above principles and are listening to God instead of the world.
- We are walking as beautiful and free women.

Working through the topics in the first four chapters of this book has been laborious, hence the reference to *working*. While the work isn't necessarily done, and I cannot promise smooth sailing from here, I can say it's about to get a whole lot more fun! The question now before us is this: what are we free to do? That is where purpose comes in.

We each have a purpose in this life, whether we've considered it or not. People want to be important and have others take notice. We struggle when we feel unnoticed. Whether it's in the company of our parents, friends, teachers, coworkers, or community, feeling unseen is not something we usually enjoy. Sometimes as women we feel we have to persist diligently to be heard and seen for those around us to notice our abilities and strengths. Even when others don't see us, God does.

The book of Samuel offers some wisdom on unrecognized purpose and potential. "But the Lord said to Samuel, 'Do not look at his appearance or his stature because I have rejected him. Humans do not see what the Lord sees, for humans see what is visible, but the Lord sees the heart'" (1 Samuel 16:7 CSB). Samuel was a prophet who was sent to anoint the next king. Above were God's instructions regarding who Samuel should select. If I were to pick someone to be the next ruler, I would want someone with experience and training. I've read and personally observed that CEOs and leaders of large companies are often tall men, and it's rare for them to be female, short, or both. I did meet a female CEO once; she was a tiny powerhouse of a woman who loved the Lord and walked with humility and grace. She treated me with respect and kindness and still made time to deliver meals on wheels. I wonder if she rose to her position because God saw her heart and made it so? God's instructions for Samuel make it clear the world may see only what is visible to them, but God sees what we cannot. The world determines qualifications based on accomplishment and training, but God qualifies those he has called and enables them to accomplish great things for him. God sees the heart and esteems the one that is after him. I believe at our core we all want to be successful, to make a difference, and to be happy, though we all have different ideas of what would constitute each of those things. God knows our heart and what it longs for. Purpose is the method God uses to satisfy our heart's desires. Samuel's purpose was to convey God's messages to the people, and David's (the one whom Samuel anointed as king) was to lead God's people. What's yours? Whether you have been walking in your purpose for years or have never considered it until this moment, we are going to walk through what every well woman needs to know about purpose.

Our Collective Purpose

In a world where competition and coming out ahead are praised and promoted, it's important to know that God's people are called to work together. My husband, like a lot of guys, is a little competitive when it comes to driving. One thing that drives him crazy is to be stuck behind a car. It's worse if said car is driving slowly, but regardless of the speed, he has a compulsive need to try to find a way around anyone who is in front of him. A saying that has become our inside joke is, "If you're not first, you're last." When I try to get him to relax and remind him that we are, in fact, driving a family SUV and not in an actual race, this is always his response to me (cue my eye roll in response to this ridiculousness). While I don't share this same need for getting ahead on the road, the saying applies to so many other areas. No matter what I accomplish, what success or happiness I experience, there will always be someone who has done or experienced something bigger and seemingly better. Again, our sinful nature has a way of sneaking in when we least expect it. I also know that women have a tendency to be snarky, and I have been on the receiving end of some unkind treatment, even in Christian circles, particularly when I was given a position someone else felt they deserved or when I accomplished something someone else desired. A good heart check for us all is to remember our collective purpose, the thing God has called us all to do together. As 1 Peter 2:9 points out, "But you are a chosen race, a royal priesthood, a holy nation, a people for his possession, so that you may proclaim the praises of the one who called you out of darkness into his marvelous light" (CSB).

As Christians we are all part of a royal priesthood, wearing those garments of salvation and robes of righteousness. We are all citizens of our own nations yet all part of God's holy nation. We belong to God and have the privilege of telling those around us about how God has called us out of darkness. We are to work together, under the same law and ruled by the same ruler, in order to proclaim God's praises. The way we each go about that will be different, but no citizen is more important than another. We are all royals, we are all his, and we all have the same end goal. Not only is what someone else accomplishes not a competition or a threat; it is a benefit to us, as it furthers our cause and brings in other priests to join us. We are in this together, and we are better when we work as a unified nation, which is how God intended.

The Great Commission (Matthew 28:18–20) may be the clearest definition of Christian purpose. Jesus tells the men who have been *his* disciples to go and *make* disciples of all nations, baptizing people and teaching them what Jesus had taught the disciples. Jesus made this statement after he lived his earthly purpose, shared his message over a lifetime, died on the cross for us, and rose from the dead. Jesus's departing words to his disciples before he left this earth tell us exactly what he wants all of us who know him as savior to do.

What does it mean to make disciples of all nations? The simplest explanation is we are to take whatever Jesus has given us and tell others. It doesn't matter if we've been a believer for a day or a lifetime—we are all commissioned. What love he has shown us we are to show others. The healing and forgiveness he has bestowed on us we are to tell others about. The knowledge we have soaked up about him we are to pour out into the world around us. Notice the significance of how Jesus told this to *all* the disciples. Each of them was important, and while they may not always work together, it was important for them to know they were all commissioned for the same purpose and had the same goals. In Scripture we often see examples of disciple teamwork, when the disciples or apostles traveled and taught together. I once listened to a teaching by Beth Moore in which she referenced how she and many other female Christian authors and speakers, all the big names many of us would recognize, are intentionally supportive of each other and actually friends. I found that to be a powerful example of the Great Commission: women who are sharing with the world what they've received from God and supporting others who are doing the same. They even team up on projects, surely bringing more people to know the Lord than they would have otherwise!

So, if you didn't know it before, I hope you are now clear on the fact that you are welcomed into the club and supported by the nation of Christians. Whether you have a team you currently work with or not, you are part of the royal priesthood. We all have the same goal: to bring praise and glory to God and to bring more people into the nation. In a world where I can easily get discouraged or feel lost, it's a comfort to know that many like-minded people in this community are not only trying to do the same thing I am, but they are usually more than willing to help me dust off my righteous robe and stay on the right path.

Your Individual Purpose

Knowing we all have a purpose, and no one has been left out, is reassuring. Realizing that being a Christian means we are part of a community purpose is inspiring and encouraging. What a well woman needs to know next is her individual calling, her way of contributing to this world and the kingdom of God. We've discussed a Christian's purpose. What we need to drill down to now is *your* purpose.

This is not a simple idea, and it's one that has taken me years to figure out for myself. In fact, my purpose is still evolving, and I believe it will continue to do so until the Lord calls me home. However, I gave absolutely no thought to purpose for many years. During those wandering years I meandered from one thing to the next, sometimes following where God graciously led despite my misguided focus and other times going where I pleased despite God calling me elsewhere. Today I have the opportunity to meet young women all the time who are so focused on God's call on their lives, intent on changing the world, and who believe they can make a difference. I was nothing like that. I wanted to do good things and help others, and I had goals professionally and personally, but there was no overarching purpose I was aiming to fulfill. As I entered my third decade, I started seeking God more and learning about who he says I am and what his plans were for me. I learned that he had a purpose for me. That knowledge alone was shocking and humbling! Who am I to deserve a God-given mission in life? I'm a daughter of the Most High King, that's who. The more I sought him, the clearer my purpose became, and I am happy to share what I've learned.

I want you to look into your heart, the one seeking after God, and make sure Satan hasn't planted any lies about your purpose. Satan will try to tell you it's too late to live your purpose; God says he's simply waiting for you to be ready. Satan will try to tell you it's too hard; God says he will strengthen you. Satan will remind you of all the ways you've messed up and squandered any chance of purposeful living; God says you are forgiven and free to become exactly who he's always known you are. If you have bought into any of those lies (like I did), soak in the knowledge that God has a purpose for you and it's time to start walking toward it.

In order to pursue purpose, we have to understand what it is. Your purpose is your God-given mission in life and the way you impact God's kingdom. We are all called to tell others about Jesus and make disciples; how you go about doing that is your purpose. It's a way of life, the goal or objective of everything you do. Purpose is how you pass along to others the love Christ has shown you.

A great example of purpose is the story of Esther. A fascinating tale in the book aptly named after the main character, the Book of Esther tells of a Jewish girl who finds herself named queen of the Persian empire. A few things are important to note about the background. First, Esther was Jewish, and at that time the Jewish people were scattered in different nations and were a powerless minority. Esther was also an orphan, raised by a cousin. Second, the reason the position of queen became available was because the king dethroned Esther's predecessor when she disobeyed him. Third, the selection process for becoming queen involved a year of beauty treatments and a trial night with the king to see if you were good enough to be chosen. My grandmother once told me, as I whined about hot rollers burning my five-year-old head, "You have to go through pain to be beautiful." I always laugh to think of that memory, but I think Esther quite literally endured some pain to be seen as beautiful enough to be queen.

All of this background, an orphaned Jewish girl's tale of a not-so-overnight rise to a most high position, happened before the climax of the story. In a strange turn of events, the king ends up being coaxed into issuing a decree to kill all Jewish people, all the while completely oblivious to the fact that Esther was a Jew herself. In a last-ditch effort to save her people, Esther finds herself considering using her position to ask the king to spare the Jews, at the risk of losing her life should he find offense with her approaching him to ask such a thing. As she considers her options, her cousin has some words of wisdom: "If you keep silent at this time, relief and deliverance will come to the Jewish people from another place, but you and your father's family will be destroyed. Who knows, perhaps you have come to your royal position for such a time as this" (Esther 4:14 CSB). I love the clarity this verse brings to the notion of purpose. Esther's purpose was not to be queen. Her purpose was to represent her people as well as God's plan for his chosen people to the non-Jewish world she was surrounded by.

Our purpose is always people centered. A Christian's general purpose is to bring glory to God and bring others to know him, and your specific purpose will be tailored to the people you are to impact. We are generally to show others the love of Christ, but you are supposed to do that in a specific way.

There are some misconceptions around the concept of purpose we need to clear up, and doing so will bring clarity to what our purpose is and identify what it's not. Esther was positioned to live her purpose, but her purpose was not her position. Our purpose is not a position or role we are in. My calling in life is not to be a nurse; it is to help others be well. My purpose is not to be a mom; it is to foster wellness in my children through showing them the love of Jesus. The roles we are in give us clues to our purpose, but they don't define our purpose, just like they don't define our identity.

Esther was noted to be beautiful, and that was a quality God used to help further his kingdom. Her beauty was not her purpose, but it was a quality God allowed to develop in her to be used for his glory. Our qualities, skills, talents, and unique traits are what God gifts us with and brings forth to allow us to live out our purpose, but they don't define our purpose. An author's ability to write isn't their purpose, but how they use that gift to impact others is likely a clue. A professional athlete's purpose is not to play a sport; it's to impact God's kingdom by how they play and how they live on and off the field. Your qualities will give you clues to your purpose by how you use them to further the kingdom of God, but they do not define your purpose.

The last misconception about purpose is perhaps the most common of all. Our culture worships achievement. The people that reach the top of their profession are often the ones we most revere. Esther's achievement of becoming queen was not the actual crowning achievement of her life; it was the beginning of God positioning her to do great things for his kingdom. God can take us to greater heights than we could ever hope or imagine, and even the greatest accomplishment would not define our purpose. We can know our purpose here on this earth, but we will never understand its true impact until we enter heaven's gates and learn of our effect on the citizens there. Oh, what a glorious day that will be! Until then, we can rest assured that the achievements God is urging us toward are not those of the world, and our purpose will never be satisfied by the awards and accolades this world offers.

If you are wondering, after all this discussion about purpose, how in the world you are going to determine what your *actual* purpose is, you've come to the right place. We know the general purpose we are all called to, and we know we each have a specific purpose to impact those around us and grow the kingdom of God. Some of us are aware of our purpose, but others aren't. No matter where you are, there are three key things a well woman needs to do to uncover, clarify, or revitalize her purpose.

First, reflect. Look back on your life thus far. What passions has God laid on your heart? Whom, or what groups of people, are you compelled to serve or reach? What are you good at? Think about both your natural talents and acquired skills. What makes your heart soar? I encourage you to make a list and look purposefully for a theme of your purpose threaded through each of these life reflections.

Second, ask God. I once was in a season of struggle with prayer. I'd had a great prayer life prior to this, one that was fulfilling and made me feel so connected to God. In my season of struggle there was a disconnect in my prayer that was so frustrating yet undeniably present. I kept trying and praying, but it didn't seem to improve. One day I was listening to the audiobook of Priscilla Shirer's *Fervent*, and she encouraged praying over your prayer life. How simply profound. If I'm struggling with anything, I should pray about it, even if the struggle is with prayer itself. So I did. I'm happy to report that after praying over my prayer life, things started to improve, and once again I was reminded of the power of prayer. If you don't know what your purpose is, or you are simply trying to get clarity around walking out the purpose you are certain you are called to, pray. Proverbs 20:5 says the heart's purpose is like deep water, but someone with understanding can draw it out. Pray for God to open your eyes, heart, and mind. Pray for him to help you discover your specific purpose. Pray for faith to believe that you have a purpose. Pray over whatever it is about purpose that is puzzling you. Then listen for the answers that will surely come.

The final step to reveal your purpose is to find community. Our purpose is people centered, and people can help us figure out what our purpose is. I think there are four groups you need to commune with: mentors, friends, mentees, and beneficiaries. Mentors are those who are a season or step ahead, able to equip and empower you. They are on a similar path and have been in a similar position as you in the past. Even if you don't know your exact purpose, you can find people who are further in their Christian walk to guide you. Look for mentors and ask them to help you. Friends are those you can relate to, who will walk alongside you and encourage you. It helps if they are doing similar things and can share in your experiences. Find a tribe, invest in them, and allow them to invest in you. Mentees are those on a similar path but a season or step behind you. No matter where you are in determining or walking out your purpose, there is someone who is coming along behind you and looking for encouragement. Look for mentees and be open to purposeful relationships with them, because a well woman is empowered by passing along what she knows. Last, find your beneficiaries, or those you intend to impact. We can't have purpose involving other people without actual people to impact. Think about those reflections on your talents and passions; whom do they impact? Whom did you think of when you reflected on the groups you are drawn to? Those are your beneficiaries. Some of us have a definite answer to this, but if it's not clear for you, just consider the possibilities and go from there. I promise, clarity will come with time.

For added reassurance, I'll share how I came to know my purpose. I already told you I spent a significant amount of time in my life purposeless. This first changed when I began to seek God intentionally. I wasn't perfect and had no idea what I was doing, I simply began to pursue him and things of him. I started attending church, serving, reading Christian books, then listening to Christian radio (but not when anyone else was in the car!). Later I kept going, opening my own Bible occasionally, and becoming more openly unapologetic about my growing faith. Eventually I wanted to join a Bible study, but the only ones at my church were during the day when I was at work. I rolled my eyes at yet another women's group that assumed no women work during the day, and wished to myself that someone would host a Bible study for women like me. That's when I heard this voice in my head saying, *you start one*. At first I ignored the voice and the ridiculous suggestion that I could do such a thing, but I could not stop thinking about it. Then I started rationalizing as to why I couldn't start a Bible study. I wasn't qualified because my Bible knowledge was, um, barely existent. I didn't have time; I worked and was going to school. I have kids who need adult supervision that I am required by law to provide. No one would want to come to a Bible study led by an unqualified introvert with a questionable background (Satan had to sneak that shame part in there). But God. While denying and questioning this calling, I felt this assurance wash over me, offering peace in the unknown. I was certain that this Bible study would happen even if I had no idea how.

Then, piece by piece, the puzzle came together. First, a friend suggested we start a Bible study. Okay. Then other friends said they'd love to join. Double okay. Then a sweet friend said she wanted to be a part but was also willing to watch kids if needed. Wow, okay then. Slowly a group of amazing sisters formed, and study by study I learned and grew along with them. One study led to another, and each step I took in faith landed me in the next position to be purposeful before I knew a single thing about purpose. Bible study led to writing, faithful steps in my career led to furthering my education, and along the way I began to see a theme emerge. In each area of my life I was impacting people similarly, though the methods I used were different and the positions I held varied. After walking obediently, I began to see connections between my steps and the impact each step had on those around me. God led me to a community that gave me the support and wise counsel I needed. My purpose wasn't an overnight revelation but a continuous evolution that was guided by trust in God who had brought me thus far. He will do the same for you, and I truly believe all he asks of us is the next step. What's yours?

There are promises throughout God's Word about purpose. Jeremiah 1:5 says we were set apart with a purpose before we were even born. Ephesians 2:10 tells us we were created for good works that God prepared ahead of time. Even if we don't know where to go or what to do with our passions, Psalm 16:11 assures us God will make the paths known to us.

Uniquely Qualified
It's important that a well woman understands she is uniquely qualified for

her purpose. David is one of the most well-known characters in the Bible. He was a shepherd boy when he was first anointed as king (which we discussed earlier in this chapter). Sometime later he famously defeated the giant, Goliath, with his slingshot. On the surface, it would seem David was no match for Goliath, since he had never been a warrior. If you looked a little deeper, you would see that David had spent years preparing for this, killing bears and lions that were coming for his sheep. The traditionally trained soldier didn't have the unique qualifications that David possessed. God may be calling you to do things that seem beyond your qualifications, but he either already has or surely will uniquely equip you to do above and beyond what you could ever imagine.

Looking later in David's story, he did become a great warrior and commander, which prepared him for his role as king. It's important to remember he was anointed many years prior, but God didn't expect him to walk in the full weight of his calling without successive steps of preparation. Our calling usually follows a similar pattern. If you have a dream, something that seems unreachable yet perfectly aligned with God's calling on your life, trust that he will guide you one step at a time in order to reach the unreachable. One final lesson from David we must remember comes from his faults. After he became king, David sinned big-time, committing adultery and even murder. Then he repented of his sins and turned back to God, and God forgave him. There were consequences of David's actions, no doubt, but he was still allowed to play a part in bringing God's presence to the world in the form of the temple and later a savior, as Jesus came through David's family line. David was not disqualified by his sins, even those he committed after he was put in position to live out his purpose in the biggest, most impactful way. God doesn't expect us to be perfect, and he honors the repentant heart chasing after him. We can never sin our purpose away.

What I notice in David's story, and my own, is a repeated pattern of God's intervention to pull us into purpose. First, there is an encounter with God; encounter is followed by a bold step in faith; the faith step results in a daily grind of sometimes monotonous details in walking out that step; eventually the daily grind unfolds into an unexpected opportunity, blessing, or healing that prepares me to take the *next* step in faith. This pattern has repeated in my life over and over, and I've come to expect and trust it. God uniquely qualifies, positions, and equips each of us to meet our purpose. Can you look back on your life and see a similar pattern? If not, pay attention going forward. Be open to encounters with God and ready to walk by faith, and expect him to be faithful to honor your steps in the most unexpected ways.

Being Purposeful

I hope at this point you've gotten some clarity around purpose and started to define God's purpose for you. Reflect, seek God, and look for your community, and the clues about your purpose will no doubt start revealing themselves. Whether we are clear on our purpose or not, we all have the opportunity to be *purposeful* right now. Simply being present in each moment, choosing to see and honor the people we are with today, is purposeful. The woman who is unclear on her purpose can take a look around and determine where she can use her gifts, talents, and passions. Maybe the best next step is to be more purposeful in caring for herself so she'll be ready to impact others in the future. We can be purposeful in our homes, jobs, churches, friendships, social media posts, or even in what we consume or purchase. Purpose can sometimes feel like a plan for the future, but I like to think of it as a guide for today. Waiting to do good things until we have absolute clarity around purpose leads to missed opportunities for meaningful connections with those around us. Be purposeful in seeking the path God is pointing you toward, and as you walk, take a look around and notice who's with you and what beauty, provision, and opportunity you encounter each day.

This daily choice to be purposeful is easier with some practical steps. If you've gotten an idea of your purpose, your God-given mission in this life, write it down. It doesn't matter how vague your understanding is at this point; write down what you know so far. I think I'm on version 7.0 of my purpose. It's okay to start with what you know and grow into a more well-defined purpose as you go. Once you've written your purpose, you need to write down goals. I think it's helpful to have a bigger goal and a smaller goal or a few of each.

Bigger goals are things that seem like dreams, far-fetched, yet something in you believes you can do it and you'd sure like to try. They are more long-term and could take years to reach. This could be anything from owning your own business to being the first woman president. It's your dream, your big goal; don't let anyone make it feel small or silly.

Smaller goals are how I define short-term goals that are often a step toward the bigger goal. This might be obtaining a degree or certification that would help you reach your big goal or doing something to prepare you for a big goal in some way. Once you have a list of smaller goals, list some specific steps you can accomplish in the next week or two to start your purposeful pursuit. I have an example of this strategy from my life so you can see what this looks like.

My purpose is to equip women to be well through the love of Jesus.

My big goal is to turn Well Woman into a ministry that truly disciples women in their walks.

A small goal is to finish this book that you are holding in your hands.

Daily steps to pursuing all of the above include writing regularly, connecting with others who write, following a daily Bible reading program, and seeking ways to disciple those around me now.

All the goals and steps I listed above are in line with my overall purpose, and writing them out helps me to see how everything connects. I encourage you to try this!

Another practical way to be a well woman with purpose is to plan ahead. I have a tendency to bite off more than I can chew, so I've learned any time I start a new goal or project to open my calendar and plan. As women we often have hidden things that are not on our calendars, like cooking dinner and family time, so don't forget to consider what unwritten obligations might be occupying that empty space in your week. Looking at the calendar and considering how much available time I have to devote to being purposeful in specific areas of my life is key to making sure I don't get overwhelmed, distracted, or discouraged. It sets a realistic tone for how quickly I'm going to make progress.

Taking time to look at your overall calendar is also a good time to evaluate the things you are doing with your time. What things are essential? What things are optional but fulfill your purpose so clearly you need to make sure they stay scheduled? What things don't align with your purpose and need to be reduced or removed? Is there space to rest? Purposeful calendar planning increases your ability to be purposeful with your days. Once you've gotten the calendar balanced and planned, pray over the activities. Everything from your morning coffee to your evening Netflix provides the opportunity to be purposeful if you invite God into it.

═══════════════

As I wrap up this discussion regarding purpose, I think it's essential to discuss how a well woman prevents growing weary of being purposeful. In the beginning, when we are starting something new and exciting and discovering our purpose, it can be exhilarating. We are energized by making new plans and feeling called to do amazing things on purpose and for a purpose that was specifically designed for us. Then the novelty wears off, and as we continue to walk this thing out, it can get tiring. At some point we will surely become discouraged. Perhaps that happens when a social media follower posts a nasty comment or when we begin to doubt our ability to make a real impact in this world. Again, Satan likes to rub salt in any little wound he can find, and he will do his best to make it big enough to stop any purposeful activity. A well woman expects fatigue and discouragement. They don't surprise her because she is prepared. Remember Deuteronomy 6:5? A well woman loves the Lord with all her heart, soul, and strength, and even if she has to go back and remember that love, she knows it's there and always makes it her motivation.

It's also a good habit to renew our minds and sense of purpose daily through prayer, and praying over Romans 12:1–2 is a great way to do this. If we offer ourselves to God daily, he will give us the discernment and motivation needed for each day. We have to keep a keen eye peeled for the things that thwart us. If we start to feel overwhelmed, that's a call to look back at that calendar and consider what's keeping us so busy, reprioritize, and remember we run our schedules, they don't run us. When we inevitably run into roadblocks, we need to pay attention. Something getting in the way of progress in our purpose may be a call to seek God's help for a way around, a heaven-sent stopping point calling us to rest a while, or a loving God preventing us from going down the wrong path. Roadblocks don't thwart us; they help us, if we are purposeful when we run into them. Even failure, though it is never pleasant at the time, can be an opportunity to learn or be restored for the well woman who is ready to rely on God. The best defense against roadblocks is an offensive approach of setting the expectation that things will get in our way. When we are falling away from God, he pursues us. When we are walking purposefully with God, expect Satan to take notice and try to get in your way. Satan will pursue you with busyness, distraction, doubt, fear, and any means he can use to stop you from bringing glory to God. Be aware, and when you recognize his work, tell him, in Jesus's name, to flee. Satan has no power we don't give him.

I have two final tactics to combat purpose fatigue. Psalm 105:4–6 tells us that as God's chosen ones we are to seek him always and remember what he has done. Sometimes the best way to re-energize ourselves when we are feeling beat down is to look back. See the things God has already done, how far he has brought us. When we are in the middle of hustling day in and day out, it's easy to miss the progress.

Look back and remember how God saved you, healed you, forgave you, and positioned you in the right place with the right people. Remember how he rescued you, comforted you, and gave you the gift of his presence during good times and bad. You can't see the finished picture—only he knows that—but you can see the threads starting to weave into a beautiful tapestry that tells the story of your life. Your purpose—a well woman's purpose—is what keeps the threads moving, and a look back helps us to know there is meaning to our purpose.

Finally, envision the future. See yourself reaching those small and big goals. Believe in God's purpose for your life, and envision yourself living it out in the most fulfilling ways you can imagine. Where you are right now is the intersection of your past and your future, and a well woman is intentional about both reflecting back and looking forward so that she is empowered to be purposeful today.

Walking in purpose, on purpose, is what a well woman does. She lives life on purpose because she loves the Lord and wants to share his love with the world—and because it's the only way she can walk with the Lord and experience him here on this earth, until she meets him in heaven. She was designed to live out the purpose that was specifically designed for her, by a loving heavenly

Father who wants not only to love, forgive, and heal her but also to fulfill her and enrich her days on this earth.

Reflection

1. What clues have you uncovered about your purpose? Hint: list your talents, roles, qualities, and passions.
2. Write out your purpose or what you think it might be if you're not sure.
3. Name one big goal and one small goal you have that align with your purpose.
4. Think about your purpose and the ways to be purposeful in day-to-day life that were discussed in this chapter. List two specific, purposeful tasks you can start today.

7 BUILDING THE TEMPLE

Learning about purpose always leaves me feeling inspired and empowered. Regardless of my background, life choices, or any physical or character trait, God says I'm accepted, anointed, and called! Unfortunately, this universal acceptance and calling is not a free pass to skip over the physical realm of this world and focus only on the spiritual. Being purposeful and living a life that honors God means caring for our physical bodies. The combination of soul and physical wellness is what the well woman is seeking to live out. It's time to shift our focus a bit to becoming mindful of our bodies, fueled by that love of Jesus and building on the foundation we've established.

Paul says, "Don't you know that your body is a temple of the Holy Spirit who is in you, whom you have from God? You are not your own, for you were bought at a price. So glorify God with your body" (1 Corinthians 6:19–20 CSB). The biblical context of this verse is a call to avoid sexual immorality, and it brings up the fascinating though somewhat confusing idea that our bodies are temples, reminding us to glorify God with our bodies. The significance of this statement is minimized if we don't go back and look at what a temple was in biblical history. The modern Christian usually attends a church of some kind, so we can relate somewhat to the idea of a building that is sacred and a place to go for worship and learning about God. Beyond that, many of us haven't experienced anything quite like the temple referenced here. In fact, the claim made by Paul to post-resurrection Christians is that *we* are now the temple.

Before we unpack the meaning of a temple, there is value in naming exactly how we see our bodies. As women we are often hard on ourselves, especially when it comes to physical appearance. With every photo I look back on, I can remember thinking about my flaws, but the woman I see looks fantastic and had no reason to feel otherwise. What about you? How do you see your body? Write in the margins a few words you use to describe it, the good, bad, and everything in between. Think of what you usually say about your body. I have come to appreciate my body, but when I consider what I say out loud about it, I realize I rarely say nice things. I am quick to talk about aches and pains, and my eyes seem ever focused on the areas I see as ugly, but I take for granted all the things this body has done over the years and miss the beautiful creation it truly is. Perhaps you can relate? By the end of this chapter I hope we acquire an understanding of what it means to be a temple and gain a rich appreciation of the temple we have been given.

The first temple was built by King Solomon, who was David's son, and was the place that God's people constructed to hold the ark of the covenant. David had desired more than anything to build the temple. He wanted to bring the once-lost ark, which represented the presence of God, back to God's people. His son, Solomon, was the one who completed the temple construction, per incredibly detailed architectural specifications. The ark of the covenant was a sacred box of sorts, which held the history of God's laws and provision for his people and reminders of God's unmatched power. Also constructed of fine materials per God's precise instructions, the ark contained the ten commandments, a jar of manna (the food God provided to Israel when they had none), and the staff of Aaron, which had budded in a divine demonstration of God's power.

Imagine how sacred some of your keepsakes are. I have a box for each of my children that contains things like the outfit they wore home from the hospital and their favorite toys when they were babies. Those boxes are precious reminders of special days that I hope never to forget. Another thing we tend to treasure are photographs. It's so special to look back on old pictures! A few years ago our car was broken into on vacation, and my laptop was among the items stolen. The laptop contained about four years' worth of family photos that I had not backed up to any other source. I cannot tell you how I grieved that loss and still get nauseated when I think of it. This kind of treasured documentation of the past is what the ark of the covenant was to God's people in Israel, and it's what the temple was built to contain and keep sacred.

Prior to the crafting of the temple was a tabernacle, a temporary pre-temple version of the Holy Place to house the ark of the covenant as God's people made their way to the promised land. Exodus 24–40 details God's instructions to Moses regarding every component of the tabernacle, from the garments worn by the priests to the placement of the ark, and these instructions offer some clarity for us about these temples we all walk around in. First, God had many contribute their time, talents, and treasures to the process of creating the temple. God had Moses ask the people to provide precious metals to be used to create the components that would go into each piece of the tabernacle, and he called on many craftsmen to use their skills to create each and every piece that would eventually be put together and used to bring God's presence to the people. I think back on my life, and I can see the influence and contributions of so many people. My parents, teachers, mentors, coaches, and friends come to mind. I can look around me right now and see how God is putting together pieces, having different people influence me in different ways to build this temple, just like he did to build the first temple and the tabernacle.

The building processes of both the tabernacle and the temple happened over a long time period. Much preparation went into the gathering of material and equipping of the builders. The process was tedious at times. There were struggles and failures along the way, like David's big ole sin that delayed the building of the temple (we mentioned this in the last chapter). Reading through the Old Testament sometimes feels like a Texas two-step. God's people take one step toward him, then follow it up with two steps back. They walk in obedience and worship God; then greed or fear take over, and they worship idols for a while. Somehow, through it all, God still managed to use these imperfect people to build his temple.

This tedious process of slowly putting together the pieces and learning from failures along the way is absolutely something a well woman can relate to. Don't mistake slow progress for no progress. Let God gather the pieces that are needed to build you up. The little details you put into every day add up to a prepared heart, mind, soul, and body that will soon be put to good use, if it hasn't already. The times we fall flat on our face are opportunities for God to pick us up. The building of a temple of God does not happen overnight, and in the process and slow progress we get to bear witness to being the beneficiary of the most masterful builder of all.

Finally, when the tabernacle was finished, it was presented to God by his people. The place that was constructed per God's instructions in order to bring God's presence to the people was offered back to God himself. God doesn't ask his people to build a temple so they can marvel at their work; he wants us to give back to him that which he has given us. The reason for this return of the creation to the creator is simple: God is never done with his people, and he always gets the glory. Once the tabernacle was completed, it became a place where God met the people. They offered sacrifices to him and came for healing there. The creation of a structure was never the point or the end goal. The point of temple building was so God could complete his work with his people and use the temple to be present with them. In the same way, we are to present our temples, in whatever stage of construction we happen to be in, back to God. He wants to work through us to dwell where we dwell and meet whom we meet. What a wonderful honor to have God's presence in us. What a marvel to represent him to those around us. It brings joy to my heart to think that every bit of detail that God put into those first temples has been put into me as well. The same is true for you. God has planned in advance the preparation and use of your temple from the top of your head to the tips of your toenails.

Knowing now what a temple is, let's give some thought to our role in the construction process. The Bible provides some insight: "Now determine in your mind and heart to seek the Lord your God. Get started building the Lord God's sanctuary so that you may bring the ark of the Lord's covenant and the holy articles of God to the temple that is to be built for the name of the Lord" (1 Chronicles 22:19). Most importantly, we have to choose, as the Israelites did, to get our direction from God. He created us and knows what is best for us. Never before have we been so inundated with sources of information on any topic, not the least of which is our health. Websites, social media, books, magazines, they are all at our fingertips. There is nothing wrong with seeking information from experts on nutrition, fitness, supplements, or any other topic. In fact, it's wise to do our homework and learn about our bodies from trusted sources. We just need to start with *the* source, who has all authority in heaven and on earth, so that he can guide us. Some ways I do this are praying before I work out, asking for God to use my health habits for his glory, fasting, and learning what God's Word has to say about our physical health. Everything I seek and learn beyond that is filtered through the lens of biblical knowledge.

Our role also involves knowing that temple building is a process, like it was for Israel. Sometimes we will be working on building up our emotional, spiritual, or mental health; other times there will be a focus on the physical. The process usually involves some demolition. We often must tear down things we've piecemealed together ourselves before we decided to seek for God's direction, removing the stuff we've been storing from past experiences. Construction may involve other skilled craftsmen (and women) whom we partner with, like the Israelites did. God gives us everyone from friends to coaches to health care professionals to help us in building up our health. It's important to know the process will be tedious at times, and temples are built by daily choices, not sudden heroic measures. We would all love to be able to buy that winning lottery ticket at the store down the road and suddenly find ourselves with full bank accounts. While some have had that happen, most don't build wealth and financial stability in a day. I've read about the high percentages of those who do receive a sudden windfall, then go on to lose every bit of that wealth in a short time. I have learned that the most effective and long-lasting benefits come from the accumulation of consistent, daily health deposits. The progress may not be visible day to day, but it's there. We can see it if we look back to the first time we said yes to God and made the choice to set our mind and heart on him. The greatest benefit of this progress is gleaned when we then offer back to God what he has done for us. Present your temple to him, ask him to use it to bring glory to him, and he will use it to shine on those around you in ways you never imagined.

God didn't create our bodies to look perfect, though he is the perfect creator. He didn't purpose them for the world to marvel at, though they are truly a marvelous wonder. Our bodies are gifts that he allows us to help build.

Our health, wherever it is today, is a blessing from God. He uses both those the world considers to be in good health and those who are currently suffering. The physical, mental, social, emotional, and spiritual abilities we have, however great or miniscule they seem, are for his glory. It's important to resist assigning value to certain traits. The world says pretty and skinny with long hair and perfect eyelashes is how all women should strive to look. I've met plenty of women who fit that description. Some are beautiful, healthy temples for God to use, and others are so lost in sickness the eye cannot see that it saddens me. Look at your body as God does, not as the world tells you. He sees your body, His creation, uniquely crafted for you, which he wants to dwell in and work through. His creations are beautiful, and you are no exception.

Look back at the words you used to describe your body. Do they align with what God says about our bodies? Does it sound like a temple made to represent him to those around you? Hopefully we've unpacked some truths that bring out thoughts about our bodies closer to how God sees them. A powerful thing to do is consider what our bodies have done for us so far. Mine has walked me to some beautiful places, allowed me to function each day, grown two live humans, and it continues to function despite some pretty questionable choices on my part at times. What has your body allowed you to do? Take a moment to be thankful for the gift of your body and a God who has brought it and you through so much to get to where you are now and still isn't done.

A well woman knows her health is both a gift from God and also her gift to offer back to him. In that offering we should consider what we can do better. If we had better habits and improved our physical well-being, how much better would that offering be? Romans 12:1–2 says we should offer ourselves as a living sacrifice every day, to a loving creator who knows exactly what we need and wants us to be well. It all starts with knowing we are a temple of the Holy Spirit, created to honor God in every way and bring glory to him. There is no shame welcome in our temples, though the Holy Spirit will certainly provide conviction for change as we go along. Love the body you have, let the Holy Spirit fill you, and watch the gradual progress from already beautiful to gloriously stunning.

Reflection

1. What is one way you bring glory to God with your body, physically, mentally, or any other way?
2. What is one daily habit you can start to ensure your temple is being built per God's specifications?
3. Name one thing you can do to represent the Holy Spirit to those around you.

8 MENDING THE MIND

Imagine a laptop with the best accessories and most advanced features but an old, worn-out processor. What about a beautifully maintained home with the best appliances, architecture, and layout but no electricity to make any of it usable. These scenarios paint a picture of what results when we care for our bodies but don't attend to our minds. Just as a computer functions only as well as the processor allows and a house is powered by electricity, we are powered by our minds.

Mental health is an essential factor of overall well-being, yet it is often pushed to the back burner. As we focus more on physical health and how we can make healthy choices that will prepare these temples to do the things we were created to do, it seems wise to start with a discussion of our minds. In health care I'm seeing a shift to focusing more on mental health. People are starting to recognize the power of a mind that is well and the struggle and suffering one experiences with mental illness. There was a time when mental illness was considered shameful, and though there is yet work to be done, we have progressed to more of an awareness and acceptance of its existence.

What a well woman needs to know is that her mind is on the forefront of her health journey. The heart and the love of God that it holds provide our motivation for seeking wellness, and the mind is what determines how we utilize that motivation. It is possible to be motivated for wellness but unable to seek it due to a mental barrier. Similar to what God does with our wounds and sins, as discussed in chapter 4, God fills in the gaps, making our minds capable of steering us to wellness. As children are growing, our culture prioritizes developing their little minds. We educate them with school, stimulate them with activities and camps, and evaluate them along the way to make sure they are progressing mentally as well as physically. Shouldn't we do the same for our own minds? As adults, the need still exists to stimulate and educate ourselves, do things that are proactively seeking mental health, and check in every now and then to make sure there isn't an unwell area that needs some attention. So, if you are like me and have not always made mental health a priority, jump in with me here, and let's learn together how to mend our minds.

The Bible has much to say about our minds. When we are made new in Christ, our mind-set changes and should be set on things above (Colossians 3:2). Sounds easy enough, but we are living in a world full of distractions, and there are numerous things pulling our minds away from that heavenly mind-set. Setting our minds on things above is a call to action that, if obediently followed, helps us to stay mentally healthy. The woman with a heavenly mind-set isn't exhausted by troubles of this world because she knows they are temporary. She prioritizes seeking things that bring her closer to God over worldly gains.

This means we sometimes turn down financial opportunities if we feel they will turn too much of our attention away from God or won't result in kingdom impact. I've read about successful entrepreneurs who have left lucrative businesses so they can pursue full-time ministry, and many women have set aside climbing the ladder of their careers out of a desire, and not a necessity, to raise and serve their families. There is nothing wrong with financial or career success, if it's where God wants you to be and you're making heaven-focused deposits. It takes a mind-set on things above to discern what is best for our eternal wellness. If you're thinking of how tough this is at times, you are not alone, and God has given us help for this particular challenge. He always equips us to do the things he calls us to. In Romans 8:5–6 the apostle Paul tells us that the Holy Spirit within us has a mind-set of life and peace, and if we live according to that Spirit, our minds will be set on the things of the Spirit. The repeated theme is to set our minds on him and things of him. God knows our affinity for distraction, and he encourages us to choose to think about him. Not only does he encourage us, but he gave us an internal guide and cheerleader to help us.

"Therefore, brothers and sisters, in view of the mercies of God, I urge you to present your bodies as a living sacrifice, holy and pleasing to God; this is your true worship. Do not be conformed to this age, but be transformed by the renewing of your mind, so that you may discern what is the good, pleasing, and perfect will of God" (Romans 12:1–2 CSB). These verses not only fall right in line with the idea that our bodies are temples, but they give us key information on how we should go about offering them to God as a sacrifice and form of worship. We have to stop conforming to the world around us, dare to be different, and by doing so allow God to renew our minds.

Have you ever had a day, week, month, or season that was mentally exhausting? I sometimes feel this way when I'm trying too hard to keep up with the world around me. Maybe I'm trying to look a certain way to fit in, work at a pace that is beyond me, or maintain near perfection in every aspect of life from the condition of my toilets to the rearing of my children. Whatever is exhausting me, the common thread is a striving for something God never asked me to seek. Exhaustion is often the result of conforming, and almost always it's a call to turn back to the only source of true renewal. Don't conform to this age. Don't get caught up in what is going on around you. Don't be pulled in a direction God doesn't intend you to go or allow yourself to be distracted by things God would never give his attention to. Don't allow the world to desensitize you or skew your view of what is right and wrong. Don't let the world tell you who you are or what you need. One key to setting our mind on him is to make sure it is not set on the world around us. Culture doesn't tell us what is acceptable, God does. Social media isn't our source of what's true, God is. The world is not the authority on how we should think, God is.

When we reject conforming, we create the opportunity for our minds to be renewed. We need to ask God to renew our minds, not every now and then but every day, because his mercies are new daily, and in this crazy world we need them as much as ever. Once we have resisted the world and allowed God to renew and transform our minds, we will then be able to discern God's will. This is where it gets interesting! Conforming to the world and allowing our minds to be polluted by things not of the Spirit will cloud our vision and hinder our judgment. Setting ourselves apart from the world and allowing God to renew our minds clears everything right up, to the extent that we can know the will of God! And his will is good, pleasing, and perfect. I want some of that; how about you?

Thus far, our approach to proactive mental health according to the Bible is as follows: have a heaven-focused mind that is guided by the Holy Spirit, avoid conforming to the world, and instead allow God to transform and renew our mind. At first this way of focusing our mind is hard, but as we practice a godly mind-set, it becomes easier over time. Eventually, it can become our natural way of thinking, and we might even start to notice how others around us could benefit from a lesson or two in not conforming. We might even be tempted to give them a piece of our mind at times, but that's where Romans 12:3 comes in. This verse reminds us that no matter how heaven-focused our minds get, we should never start to think too highly of ourselves. A renewed mind needs to remain a humble one that seeks wisdom and cherishes understanding (Proverbs 19:8), while remembering the source of all wisdom is still on the throne, and we are not yet seated with him. Our mental health is affected greatly by the gift of humility. Remember that mental exhaustion? One who thinks highly of themselves has the impossibly tiring task of trying to maintain the facade of being wise in all things, while the humble are free to mess up and seek a new opportunity for renewal every day.

Take time to set your mind on things above, let the Spirit guide you in doing so, remain humbly obedient to the source of all wisdom, and you will be a woman on the right track for excellent mental health. It's also important to know that while this preparation is important and beneficial, it's certainly not a guarantee that you will never encounter mental health struggles. At one time or another we will all suffer, as the Bible warns us, and mental suffering is no exception. We've already discussed fatigue or exhaustion, which is a form of mental suffering. Other mental struggles include stress, anxiety, fear, despair, and mental illness. According to the National Institutes of Health, 22.3 percent of American women, over 46 million, live with mental illness.[iii] Here are some additional statistics:

- Only about half of those people have received mental health services of some sort in the last year.[iii]
- Depression is one of the most common mental illnesses, again higher in women, and only 35 percent of those who'd had a major depressive episode received any treatment.[iv]
- Over 30 percent of American adults experience anxiety at some point in their lives.[v]

What's the point? Glad you asked. We need to know that many of us, if not all of us at one time or another, have some form of mental illness. That means if you are one of those many who are currently or have previously experienced mental illness, you are not alone in that suffering. Unfortunately, of those who do have mental illness, very few are getting help from professionals, perhaps partly due to feeling helpless, embarrassed, or even ashamed. Despite the stigma, mental illness is not shameful, any more than high blood pressure or arthritis is. Despite the fear and doubt, there absolutely is help for mental struggles and illness.

How can we do with our mind what God's Word says despite our mental struggles? This is a powerful question for all of us to consider. Romans 8:28 assures us that God works "all things" for our good, and it seems mental struggles would fall under the category of "all."

The question of how to be well even though we struggle with mental health is one I've had to wrestle with myself. I suffer from anxiety, though many would not know that by looking from the outside. My anxiety doesn't cause much in the way of outward signs; it's more of a burden that I hold on the inside, and at times it has tried to destroy me. Mental illness feels like a betrayal of the very vessel that is supposed to carry us through this life. It causes our physical body to react in ways that we feel powerless to stop and sometimes even mistake as other issues. So often, people with mental health struggles come to me in the clinic because they have physical symptoms of their mental distress, and it wasn't until those outward, physical signs showed up that they became concerned. In fact, we are often convinced that the harm mental illness inflicts on our bodies is due to something else. Personally, anxiety has caused me to experience headaches, stomach upset, forgetfulness, chest pain, and much more. These could be symptoms of many things, but to assume they are due to a physical disease as opposed to a mental one is misguided and keeps us ill. I had to go through a process of naming anxiety as my particular issue, and learning to cope with that anxiety, to become well even while having a mental struggle.

The process for being mentally well despite having mental challenges is very similar to the process of healing discussed in chapter 3.

First, in order to enable our minds to be set on God, we need to identify what our mental struggles are. Remember those hackberry trees? Sometimes they have been growing a while and stand taller than the healthy plants, and other times they are underneath the surface and not easy to uncover. Sometimes we see our struggles clearly, and other times we have a hard time recognizing them for what they are. There are three ways I know of to identify mental health struggles, and it should come as no surprise that the first method is prayer. Whether you know your mind is weary or you feel mentally sound at this moment, I would challenge you to pray for God to reveal your mental health issues. Acknowledge that he is Lord over you, including your mind, and that he sees what we cannot. God will make known what needs to be known, when the time is right, and what I have experienced is he often waits for me to ask. Pray for God's help in discerning your mental health struggles.

The next way to identify mental health struggles is through professional help. God has given us the gift of people he has prepared to help us in many ways, mental health professionals included. There are psychiatrists, psychologists, counselors, therapists, and probably many more trained professionals all equipped to help us identify what the problem is. Your primary care provider is a great place to start and can be a valuable resource. We don't have to figure it out alone, and it's a whole lot easier if we don't. If you are not sure you've discerned exactly what your mental health issues are, get help today.

The third way to identify mental health struggles is to ask for help from the people who know and care about you. This is one we have to be careful about, as well-meaning friends can sometimes mistake their google search for a medical degree, and even the sweetest most humble of friends can sometimes use the wrong words. Still, I encourage you to ask a trusted friend or family member to help you identify your mental health struggles. Ask questions and listen to their responses. Share with them your fears, anxieties, and general thoughts, especially if you are feeling mentally ill or exhausted. Ask them to pray for your mental health and even to pray *with* you about your mental health. Be honest about your thoughts and mind-set as well as open to their sincere concerns and observations that you may not be able to see from your perspective. Our friends and family may not have the ability to diagnose mental illness, but they very likely can offer clues to our struggles that we can use, along with prayer and professional help, to identify issues so that we can begin to walk in mental wellness despite our struggles.

After identifying our mental health struggles, we need to acknowledge their existence and then release them to the capable hands of our Father, like we did with our sin and our wounds. Acknowledging that a mental health issue exists is powerful, and acknowledging that we are not capable on our own to overcome it is key. When it comes to mental illness—more than most other types of illness, it seems—we tend to want to overcome the issue on our own. We might be resistant to help of any kind, thinking we can simply will ourselves to be well. Can I be frank for a moment? It does not work that way. I'll take it one step further and say that even if you are able to overcome a mental illness on your own for a time, it will eventually rear its ugly face again, leaving you feeling even more defeated and perhaps completely devastated.

Humility is key in this acknowledgment and release process. The fact that we have mental issues or illness does not mean we are weak; it means we are human, like every other person on God's green earth. Give yourself permission to be human, and take hold of the power that comes with naming your struggle and acknowledging it exists. Then give it to God. In Matthew 11:28–30 Jesus invites us to give our burdens to him so that we can rest. Just like we did with our sins and wounds, release your mental health struggle into his capable hands. Finally, tell someone else about your struggles and what you are acknowledging and releasing. We were made to be in community, and there is hope and support to be found in speaking out loud what you are going through. Perhaps talk to the same person you asked to help in identifying the issue in the first place. Share with your best friend, spouse, or another trusted friend or family member. Consider finding a support group or community that you can relate to. I have never regretted speaking my struggles out loud to people who cared about me, I have always been thankful I did.

Finally, once we've identified the mental health struggle, acknowledged and released it to God, it's time to seek healing. Once God's carrying the load, we may need to soothe some sore muscles or rub salve on our saddle sores from the miles we carried that load ourselves. The steps for seeking healing are a repeat of the steps for identifying struggles: pray, get professional help, and get help from your community. Once we know what the mental health issue is and we've given it to God, we need to seek his guidance, as well as that of professionals, to walk in healing. Through prayer and professional help we can become equipped and able to set our minds on him and be mentally well despite having even significant mental health struggles. Our community, whether it's those in our close circle of loved ones or a group that shares in our lived experience, can also help to equip us through listening, empathy, sympathy, and sharing their own experiences. Knowledge and acknowledgment are powerful, but healing only comes if we choose to walk fully in it, embracing the help we are so mercifully given.

There are some common mental health strategies, which both help prevent mental struggles and help address mental illnesses of many kinds, that I wanted to include as a practical tool in this chapter. There are some essential areas we need to focus on to ensure we are enabling ourselves to set our minds on God and receive transformation.

Rest and Sleep

First, we need to ensure adequate sleep. We will get into the details of both rest and sleep in the next chapter, but for now I simply wanted to make sure we are aware of the significant impact sleep has on our minds. Without sleep, we have difficulty concentrating, making decisions, and learning. Most adults need seven to nine hours of sleep, and if that's not what you are getting, this is an issue.[vi] Mental illnesses are often negatively impacted by poor sleep, as is overall mental health. So, if you have work to do with your sleep, hang on for more information in the next chapter.

Activity, Exercise, and Sunshine

Physical activity and exercise are significant contributors to mental health and overall wellness. Studies have shown that exposure to greenspace is associated with lower levels of depression, anxiety, and stress[vii] and that physical activity outdoors is associated with greater reductions in depression and anxiety than physical activity indoors.[viii] More recently, blue space (e.g., waterfront spaces) has been associated with higher well-being, further suggesting that nature may be important.[ix] Being active and exercising is about more than our physical bodies; it's good for the mind as well. Get outside as much as you can for some sunshine and move around. Personally, I find outdoor exercise to be a good time to set my mind on God. Being with him, surrounded by the beautiful things he's created, is the perfect way to focus on him and things of him.

Food

Diet is another strategy we will chew on in the next chapter, but I wanted to touch on it here in relation to mental health. A diet high in sugar and carbohydrates can cause fatigue and negatively affect mood. Eating a variety of vegetables, fruits, proteins, and healthy fats nourishes our minds as much as our bodies. I'm not aware of a diet to prevent mental illness entirely, but I know there is significant evidence that a healthy diet can help to manage the symptoms of mental illness and help us to feel better and think more clearly. We need to make good food part of our mental health plan.

Mental Stimulation

Another strategy for mental health is making sure we are engaging our minds. The fact that the Bible tells us to set our minds indicates we have a choice in what we think about. I am not a slave to my mind, and the Holy Spirit enables me to choose what I think about. Part of making choices is intentionality. Like a classic car, our minds work better when put to good use and taken through the paces on a regular basis. When overworked, the same car becomes worn and starts to break down, yet with the right blend of regular use, rest, and maintenance it can perform to its full potential. Our minds need to be used regularly in order to keep them functioning well. I do this by engaging with the people around me and continuously learning how to help others to be well. Reading, writing, and pursuing any type of learning are my methods for mental maintenance. You might enjoy creating, drawing, or organizing. Find ways to stimulate your mind regularly.

Mindfulness

It's easy and normal to react to our current situation. Most of us also find ourselves dwelling on the past or thinking about the future. Reflection can be helpful, and dreaming of tomorrow is often fun and inspiring, but a mental focus that is anywhere but in the present is likely to be mentally draining or even distressing. Mindfulness is an awareness of our present state and an acknowledgment of our feelings and thoughts without judging them as right or wrong.[x] Known to reduce stress, anxiety, depression and even pain as well as to improve quality of life, mindfulness can be practiced by meditating or practicing deep breathing while intentionally being attentive to our thoughts.[x] If you often struggle with letting your thoughts overwhelm you, try learning more about this technique. We have the choice to set our minds on things above. An awareness of what is on our minds at each moment is a powerful tool to utilize in making sure our minds aren't distracted or pulled in an earthly direction.

Professional Guidance

Last though certainly not least, an underutilized strategy for mental health is professional help. We've already touched on how mental health professionals can help us identify and name our mental struggles, but their skills and knowledge can do much more than diagnose. Professional help can equip us to be mentally well by providing us with the benefit of knowledge and expertise from an impartial third party. Professional guidance includes everything from counseling to interventional techniques, sometimes including medications. I'd like to take a moment to dwell on medicine for a moment, especially as it relates to mental illness. I find that people are often opposed to taking medications for a mental health diagnosis. While I can understand the concern, I feel it is often misguided.

Consider for a moment that you found yourself suffering from a physical injury. Let's say you are a middle-aged woman who set out to play in your local coed softball league, and in a moment of glory you slid into home plate, scoring the winning run! Unfortunately, you are not a professional athlete, and your not-so-graceful slide resulted in tearing one of the ligaments in your knee. First of all, as soon as you realize the knee was hurting, I bet you'd take notice and start looking for relief. You would probably ice and rest it, propping it up to prevent further stress and injury. Pretty soon, you'd decide to go see a professional and get the knee checked out. Bummer, the doctor says you need to have surgery. Once the surgery is completed, there is healing and physical therapy. While healing and working on strengthening your muscles and joint, I bet you'll take some medicine for pain. That medicine doesn't make the healing joint instantly better, but it does enable you to tolerate the work needed to get functional again.

What this example points out is that we are much more likely to seek professional help and accept recommended interventions for a physical problem, yet we hesitate to do the same for mental issues. Medicine isn't always the answer, but it can lessen the suffering of mental illness, and it is sometimes as essential to a person with mental illness as insulin is to a diabetic. Seek mental health professionals for help, and be open to collaboration with them to develop a plan to improve your mental health.

While the world sometimes sweeps mental health under the rug, God made it a priority to give us instructions for setting our minds on him. There is help for being mentally well, and a well woman chooses a heaven-focused mind-set, equipped by pursuing mental health.

Reflection
1. Think about what occupies your mind. List the top three things that you think about.
2. Stress, anxiety, depression, fear, and many other mental struggles make having a heavenly mind-set challenging. What is your most common mental health struggle?
3. Of the strategies listed in the chapter, what is one thing you can start doing to set your mind on God, despite your mental health issues?

9 NOURISHING THE BODY

If there are sweets in my house, I find it incredibly hard to resist them. I can't tell you how many times I've baked a pan of brownies "for the kids" only to eat half the pan myself. I almost immediately regret that choice. It's not usually the guilt or shame, nothing quite that deep. The regret comes on as my stomach bloats and cramps and physical misery sets in. I've never had that same type of regret from a sensible salad or balanced meal of protein and colorful vegetables. I feel great after those! The things we see that look so tempting and instantly satisfy our superficial cravings almost never nourish us for the long term. Instant satisfaction usually works that way: it leaves as quickly as the temptation comes.

I have a shirt that says "Remember Your Why," and this is a fantastic time for us to do that. We can probably all agree that most of us want to live a long life, and we would like to be healthy enough to enjoy it. While seeing my grandkids grow up is motivating, somehow I forget all about those unborn whippersnappers when I see that yummy pan of brownies. That's why we have to "remember our why." The long-lasting motivation for making healthy choices is our all-consuming, wholehearted love of the God who loves us. When we choose to love God every day, a love of ourselves is sure to follow. When I open my Bible out of a love for God, I'll find truths about his love for me. As I draw nearer to him, it becomes easier to love and care for myself and much harder to make bad choices. The result of remembering our "why" and walking it out in our daily choices is the step-by-step construction of one amazing temple.

Nutrition

"Why" is the perfect place to start, and points us in the right direction. To get a little more practical, nutrition is the first answer to how we nourish our bodies. In Genesis 3, the very first book of the Bible, Satan used food to tempt Eve. That crafty serpent offered her an apple, and she couldn't resist.

I could spew some harsh judgment and tell you how wrong it is to partake in the things God has clearly told us not to, except I already told you about my weakness for brownies. Just like Eve and her apple, I let temptation get the best of me. I bet you can relate. Maybe your temptation isn't forbidden apples or brownies. Whatever it is, take a minute to think about what leads you to make poor dietary choices. Genesis 3:6 tells us Eve thought the tree of life was "delightful to look at, and that it was desirable for obtaining wisdom" (CSB). Sometimes our eyes betray us, and we see things as delightful and desirable because we are being fed deceptive lies. Cravings, emotions, addictions, stress, and the simple fact that I enjoy the taste of certain foods are all things that lead me to eat things that are bad for me. Lack of planning, the convenience of unhealthy foods, and going for low cost over high value are big contributors to my poor dietary choices as well. I'm guessing you can relate to some of these, and maybe you can think of other factors that encourage your bad nutritional choices. Whatever they are, it's helpful to name and acknowledge our temptation factors so we can be prepared to resist temptation in the future.

What are the consequences of our poor diet choices? That list could be endless. Some things that come to mind are weight gain, bloating, fatigue, feelings of guilt, cardiovascular diseases, and digestive issues like diarrhea or constipation (sorry, I'm a nurse, I had to mention it!). The most important consequence we don't necessarily see with our eyes is that our body cannot be the temple it was created to be. Eve's poor choice caused her path in life to change course, and the life she and Adam led after that choice was different than what God intended. Genesis 3 outlines the consequences of this very first sin, and perhaps the most significant was the distance it put between man and God. Sin always distances us from God, and any choice that goes against what God says is good for us is sin, and our choices can alter our course and take us places God never wanted us to go. The good news is God always has a plan for redemption, and he gave us Jesus. Nothing we do changes God's love for us, and he never stops waiting for us to turn back to him.

No matter what body you were given or where you are now physically, we can start to make choices that bring us back toward, or help us become more of, the person that we were created to be. While forgiveness frees us from the consequences of sin, that forgiveness doesn't necessarily eliminate those consequences. While we can't eliminate overnight the consequences of years of poor eating, we can begin to make choices that honor the body God gave us as the temple that he intends it to be. Whether we've made good nutritional choices for years or we're starting today, God will honor those obedient choices.

Daniel 1 tells a tale that is rich with helpful instructions on how to make good dietary choices and offers so much hope in their benefits. The setting is Babylon after the Israelites had been taken captive by the Babylonian king. In the story Daniel and three of his friends are among the Israelite men chosen by the king to be trained to fill a few select spots as his servants. Think assistant to a celebrity or the right-hand (wo)man to the president; this was a big deal.

Daniel and the other candidates were to spend three years in training, learning the language and literature, eating their daily provisions, and drinking their assigned wine per the king's instructions. "Daniel determined that he would not defile himself with the king's food or with the wine he drank" (Daniel 1:8 CSB). In fact, he was so determined that he made his intentions clear. I love the way he went about following his convictions. So often in today's world we are intolerant of each other's beliefs and lifestyles, but not Daniel. He had been raised on a Jewish diet and wasn't about to conform to go against what he knew to be a healthy way to eat, but he also wasn't the kind of guy who limited what God could do with him because of his arrogance. He humbly sought to follow his convictions by asking for permission to follow his own diet: "So he asked permission from the chief eunuch not to defile himself" (Daniel 1:8 CSB). This was a bold move because if the king got wind of this and was angry, Daniel could have been killed. The text tells us God granted Daniel favor with the eunuch, even though the eunuch was worried what would happen to him if Daniel's diet caused him to be too thin.

Good thing Daniel's diet worked out. In fact, after a ten-day trial period Daniel and his buddies looked so much better than the rest of the guys that the eunuch decided it was fine for them to eat how they saw fit. It's interesting how all the other men who were training with Daniel and his friends didn't join in on their diet at this point or that the eunuch didn't tell the king about this amazingly effective diet so they could have all the men be strong and healthy. Sometimes even when we have good examples and are equipped to do better, we continue to do things the same way we have been doing them. The story says, following Daniel and his friends' faithfulness and commitment to healthy habits, God gave the four young men incredible knowledge and understanding. Daniel had an additional gift of interpreting dreams, and he and his friends were selected to stay and serve the king, being consulted often by the king for their wisdom.

We all know eating healthy benefits our physical bodies. In Daniel's case, these benefits were so vast and noticeable that he stood out and even appeared healthier than those around him. A healthy diet helps us to feel better, and often those small everyday choices show in how we look. The other interesting benefit, according to this story, is that Daniel's obedience in something as seemingly nonspiritual as his diet led to God gifting him with abilities and positioning he wouldn't have obtained otherwise. Now, I've eaten my fair share of greens and whole grains and have yet to be given supernatural powers. We learn from biblical stories by observing God's character in them and noticing the way he works. This story seems to tell us that the more we honor God with our bodies, the more he is able to entrust to us. It's not only about looking good and feeling great; it's about being fueled and nourished so that we are ready to walk into what God has for us.

If you're like me, you're pumped right about now. We all want to look great, feel great, and, by God, do great things! But how? How do we make good nutritional choices with so many options and temptations out there?

Let me first encourage you with a few powerful verses:
- "So, whether you eat or drink, or whatever you do, do everything for the glory of God" (1 Corinthians 10:31 CSB).
- "The Lord commanded us to follow all these statutes and to fear the Lord our God for our prosperity always and for our preservation, as it is today" (Deuteronomy 6:24 CSB).
- "If you find honey, eat only what you need; otherwise you'll get sick from it and vomit" (Proverbs 25:16 CSB).

Motivation, preservation, and moderation are the key instructions in these verses. We should eat in a way that aligns with our motivation that comes from loving Jesus with everything we've got, including the nutritional choices we make. The foods we eat should not only be God-honoring for eternity; they should sustain us and preserve us for today. Too much of even a good thing will be bad for us, so we've got to keep our indulgences in check.

Living this out is better done with some basic nutritional knowledge. Two topics I think are helpful to familiarize yourself are calories and nutrients. Calories are the unit of measure that represents how much energy a food contains. Our bodies require caloric intake to function, and we burn calories simply by existing at what is referred to as our basic metabolic rate. Activity increases how many calories we burn and therefore requires more caloric intake. Most women require 1,200 to 2,000 calories per day, and that number varies based on age, weight, height, activity level, and other factors. It's important to know how many calories you should aim for, and it can be enlightening to track your calories. There are several apps you can use to do this, and they provide accountability, helping you stay within your calorie goal and learn to make better choices. Fun fact about calories: it takes a deficit of 3,500 calories to lose a single pound! Tracking calories is helpful for weight loss because it allows you to create that deficit in small increments every day. Even if you're not trying to lose weight, knowledge of calories gives you power because it equips you to eat the right amount of food.

Nutrients, the other main nutritional concept I recommend considering daily, are the components of food that nourish us. All food is not created equal, and you want the calories you consume to offer a variety of nutrients. Macronutrients are the categories used to define the three essential types of calorie sources: carbohydrates, proteins, and fats. The Institute of Medicine generally recommends we get 45–65 percent of our calories from carbohydrates, 10–25 percent from protein, and 20–35 percent from fat.[xi] Though there are a plethora of options for diets or nutrition plans, I would simply say it's important to get a balance of macronutrients to fuel our bodies adequately. It's also important to eat a variety of naturally occurring fruits, vegetables, and proteins in order to get the proper mix of vitamins and minerals, which are referred to as micronutrients.

Getting the right amount and types of food in our diets is essential for our health, and doing so helps us to feel well and live as well women. If you're ready to make healthier dietary choices, I'd start by taking an inventory of what you eat now. It's very helpful to download an app and record everything you take in for a week or so, then see how the numbers shake out. If you're lacking any nutrients or your calorie count is off one way or the other, it'll show and you'll usually be able to see where you're going wrong. Knowing what you're doing wrong is key to figuring out how to do better. Notice the focus on what you need to eat versus focusing on what you can't have. When we want to lose weight or even maintain a healthy weight, I find it so helpful to identify what you should be eating and find options in that category that you will enjoy. Eating healthy is about nutrition and nourishment, not deprivation and starvation.

I also think a healthy diet is only as good as the planning and preparation put into it. As women motivated by a love of Jesus to love our bodies well, it's important to invest some time and thought into how we fuel that body. Do some meal prep, plan your grocery list around recipes, make a meal calendar, and put the pieces into place that set you up for dietary success. Avoid poor choices that result from poor planning, like the fast food runs that happen when you don't take a snack during errands or a lunch to work. Be like Daniel: commit and reap the benefits that will undoubtedly follow.

Activity

When most of us think of health and wellness, exercise is one of the first things that come to mind. Some view exercise as essential, some enjoy it, some trudge through it because they know it's good for them, and others view it as a dirty word. I think it's important to take a minute to evaluate your current level of activity by asking yourself a few questions.

- On a scale from zero to ten, how important is exercise to you?
- How many minutes per day are you moving and active?
- How many minutes per day do you participate in vigorous

exercise that increases your heart rate?
- How many minutes per day are you sitting or sedentary?
- What type of exercise do you enjoy most?

Hold onto those thoughts as we see what the Bible has to say about physical activity.

Training to be godly is beneficial in every way, and training our bodies also has benefits that, while not as significant as learning to become more like Jesus, are still valuable (1 Timothy 4:7–8). We've already established our body as a temple, so it follows that training it to be fit for the job is clearly important.

The apostle Paul wrote, "So I do not run like one who runs aimlessly or box like on beating the air. Instead, I discipline my body and bring it under strict control, so that after preaching to others, I myself will not be disqualified" (1 Corinthians 9:26–27 CSB). I discipline my body so I am more able to reach others. I discipline my body with a purpose so that I can live life on purpose and live out *my* purpose. God's Word gave us this encouragement to be disciplined, and exercise is one way to do so. Now, this doesn't mean we are not qualified to disciple others if we aren't thin enough or perfectly healthy. God qualifies the ones he calls, and he's the only judge of what we are qualified to do. This verse is referencing self-control and training ourselves for a heavenly prize in the way an athlete trains for a prize. I'm simply calling our attention to physical activity as a form of self-control and a means of seeking to be more godly, more like a temple fit for the King. There is no shame if your temple needs some touching up; mine does too. But let's be committed enough to live out our faith physically as well as spiritually; let's be disciplined in submitting ourselves as a living sacrifice that is pleasing to God (Romans 12:1).

The benefits of physical activity on our bodies are vast. We discussed how exercise is associated with better mental health; it also improves our cardiovascular health and helps us maintain a healthy weight, which in turn decreases our risk for everything from depression to diabetes. As we age, exercise becomes important to maintain healthy bones and muscle mass, decreasing our risk for falls and injuries. One of the key gains gleaned from a lifestyle that includes regular exercise is simply improved quality of life. I feel better when I exercise, I'm physically more able to do things I enjoy, and I'm happier with the woman I see in the mirror. At one point I decided I was too busy to exercise and no longer needed to go to the gym like the twenty-somethings. It didn't take long for me to notice how breathless I got going up stairs and how my pants were getting tighter. Then I read an article geared toward women my age encouraging us to shift from a mind-set of exercising as a means to be thin to one of exercising to stay healthy as we begin to age. It was my first realization that the time I spend in the gym or walking my dogs is time invested in my future self. No matter what, we are not promised tomorrow, but if we are given the gift of another day, we will certainly be better able to enjoy it if we are physically capable of doing so.

Wherever you landed with your assessment of your own physical activity, think about how you train to be godly; then make a plan to ensure you are physically capable of showing the world what God has done for you and is doing through you. Generally, most recommendations are for at least 150 minutes of moderate-intensity activity per week. If you're not getting in that much, how can you work your way toward that? If you need to improve in this area, make one or two realistic goals for yourself. Commit to exercising at least three times per week if you're starting out, or make a goal to work your way into walking or running a certain distance. Joining a gym is not a goal. Goals are specific and measurable. Commit to running a certain number of miles per week, attending a specific number of exercise classes per month, and so on. Then do it. Give yourself something you can work toward, and then once you crush that goal, make a new one! If you loathe exercise and find yourself sedentary more than you should be, I would not encourage you to take on an exercise routine you hate. Find an activity you enjoy, and find ways to be more active throughout the day. Take the long walk to the break room at work, park farther away when you grocery shop, take the stairs every chance you get, and simply move more. Remember your "why": because you love Jesus and he loves you and wants you to be well!

Rest

When I say rest, I'm usually referring to two main topics: Sabbath rest and sleep. Both are essential, and they are related to one another, though each is unique in what it requires.

The first mention of Sabbath rest in the Bible is when God himself rests from all the creating he did in the beginning of time (Genesis 2:2). The thing is, God doesn't get tired. He's God. So I have to think he rested for other reasons. For starters, the word used for *rest* means to cease or stop, which would lead us to believe it was more about the absence of work than taking a nap. He had created all that was needed, and it was time to stop. It also seems like this was a great way to lead by example, because if God felt the need to rest, we certainly should recognize that need for ourselves and do as he did. Rest also became part of God's covenant obligations for the Israelite people, right up there with sacrificing to atone for sin (Exodus 34:21), and God even told the people that his presence with them would give them rest (Exodus 33:14). Sometimes we think of these Old Testament commands as old-fashioned, and we write them off as things we are no longer required to do. Jesus certainly came and mercifully atoned for our sin, relieving us of the need to sacrifice in atonement, and he came to give us life everlasting with the Father. Jesus did not change the character of God, nor his heart for his people. God created us and knows what we need, and rest is a good thing for us still today. Hebrews 4:8–11 reminds us of the need to rest, even pointing out that not resting remains an act of disobedience that can lead us to sin because we're not prepared to make good choices. When unrested, I will snap at my husband or children more often, and tend to over-eat. Disobedience of any kind is always an opportunity to enter a sin cycle, and choosing not to rest has sent me spinning many times. I'm learning to stop the cycle by prioritizing rest.

My tendency is to power through and work until I can't keep going, stepping over this command to rest like it's a penciled-in request God wasn't serious about. But it wasn't penciled in; it was set in the same stone tablets as the other nine commandments. My clues that I've put off rest for too long are exhaustion, excess stress, and hitting walls I can't seem to get past. Rest not only gives us a break; it gives us the opportunity to see what all we've done and recognize God's work in and through us. More than that, Sabbath rest provides restoration as we lean into God as our one true source of strength.

If you don't know where to start with making rest a priority, Matthew 11:28 tells us to simply come to him, and he will literally give us rest. Carve out time to sit with God and do nothing else. Work your way into setting aside a whole day. The Jewish tradition is to rest from sunset on Friday night until sunset Saturday, and the Jews take it seriously. I've read that Friday afternoons in Israel are bustling with activity as people prepare for Sabbath. In American culture we like to hustle, and there's nothing wrong with that when the time is right. God called on people to hustle all throughout biblical history. But he also called us to rest, and I love the idea of hustling into rest. Be intentional about planning for rest, and do what needs to be done as you prepare for your Sabbath. Then when Sabbath comes, rest in him, doing things that draw you into his rest. For me that includes spending time with family, praying in solitude, doing outdoor activities, and going to church. It does not include hours of scrolling through social media or doing housework, both of which distract me from things that are godly and good. I've already confessed my struggle with this, but I'm trying, and you should too.

If rest is how our soul recharges, sleep is how our physical body does the same. Getting seven to nine hours of sleep nightly improves mood and concentration and is physically required for our bodies to be able to do what we need them to do. Sometimes I want to stay up late to get work done, and as I become more and more tired, I find it harder and harder to accomplish anything. After a good night's sleep, those same tasks that seemed so hard are suddenly so much easier to complete. It's amazing what sleep does for us! It's almost as if we were designed for it to be part of our day.

Just like you did for nutrition and exercise, think about your habits around rest and sleep, and consider how you can be more intentional with both of them. How can you ensure the week doesn't carry you away and you plan for a time of rest? If you're not getting adequate sleep, make it a priority to do better.

Sometimes sleep habits are the problem and you're not setting yourself up for a good night's sleep, and other times we need to seek professional help in this department. Being aware sleep is an issue is the first step toward fixing the problem, and solutions usually make themselves clear to the person willing to acknowledge the problem and seek to do better.

Good nutrition, an active lifestyle, along with adequate sleep and rest are ways we live out our "why." It's not enough to say we love Jesus; we have to live like it. Part of that head-over-heels love for Jesus is daily walking like we love ourselves the way Jesus does. We can all do this better. Wherever you see room for improvement in nourishing your temple, don't let that awareness fizzle into something you should have done but never got around to. Make a specific goal to address at least one area and a plan to reach that goal with daily habits. If diet is a struggle for you, challenge yourself to stop one unhealthy habit and start eating better. Plan to start each day with a healthy breakfast, or drink at least a hundred ounces of water per day, for instance. God doesn't expect perfection, but I believe he does expect effort.

Nourish and nurture yourself well so you will be well enough to be the woman he already sees you as.

Reflection
1. Write one specific goal to address your physical health.
2. List one or two daily habits you plan to start in order to progress toward that goal.
3. Who or what would enable you to reach your goal? For example, if you want to exercise more, having a friend to walk with might be helpful.

10 NURTURING THE SOUL

For the first decade or so of my adult life I placed a high priority on physical health. My profession was centered around it, and my personal life prioritized healthy cooking and regular exercise. I've always seen the benefits of maintaining a healthy body because I've spent so much time caring for people who didn't do so.

The first time it occurred to me that I might want to focus more on soul care was when I was pregnant with my first child. Early in the pregnancy I had what's referred to as a threatened abortion, which is unfortunately quite common and likely has happened to many reading this book. I began bleeding, and it scared me. Looking back, what was perhaps more concerning is that I was completely unprepared to deal with this spiritually. I remember being suddenly aware of how little I prayed in my daily life, feeling like now was too little, too late. I thought, "How can I ask God to help me now when I don't even talk to him regularly?" Of course, I now know that is one of Satan's tools, to use any opportunity to discourage us from calling on God and shame us into distancing ourselves further. God will convict us to turn to him, never shaming us or pushing us further away. It's never too late to turn to God if there is still breath in our lungs, and God is never disappointed to see the face of his child looking at him. While it was more than acceptable for me to seek God in my hour of need, I would have been better prepared to do so if I had invested some time in regular soul care. It often takes a low point in life to get us to look up. The truth, whether we realize it yet or not, is that we need God and we always will.

I was once talking to a patient about his smoking, encouraging him to stop this unhealthy habit. I asked him how much he was smoking, and his reply stuck with me. "Just one at a time," he replied. I chuckled. I also couldn't help but think of how profound that response was and how applicable it is to any habit. Bit by bit, regular habits have the power to help or harm us. No one would consider taking in a lifetime of smoke exposure in one breath, but many breathe it in slowly day after day, hardly noticing the damaging effects until they are irreversible and devastating. The same can be true of growing in our relationship with God. We aren't capable of taking in all that he is and everything he has to offer in one breath, but we can develop a relationship that will nourish our souls for a lifetime with daily investment.

What does regular nurturing of our souls look like? I think there are five ways of doing this, each of which we've already touched on throughout this book. I'd like to take a moment to weave them together into practical application for regular soul care. In fact, I want to empower you to weave a tapestry of daily investment in your soul that will enable you to be well on the brightest days or darkest nights.

Time with God

The first essential for soul care is regular time with God. This comes in many forms but, most importantly, must include you spending time engaged with the Father. This is not necessarily the time you spend at church or that amazing ladies' event you attended last summer, though those can be soul nourishing as well. What I'm referring to is one-on-one time with God. We can do this in several ways. Prayer, reading the Word, and simply sitting with him are all options. Certainly, God speaks to us directly at times during group events, but I believe he desires to be the center of our attention, alone with us.

Walking this out day after day, week after week, year after year is what helps us hear him more clearly and feel his presence in our lives more palpably. The best way to hear him is to listen (see chapter 4), so I try to make regular practice of doing this, though being silent is a challenge. I tend to want to do the talking, as many of us do.

Perhaps listening isn't your struggle, but you have a hard time reading the Bible. I hope the discussion in chapter 4 helped you feel more confident in getting into the Word. It's so beneficial to make time for God every day. What this looks like for me varies, but generally, mornings are my Jesus time. Most weekdays I start the day with a prayer on my way to work out. After I work out, I spend time reading my Bible before taking a shower and getting on with my day. Sometimes I miss the Bible reading for one reason or another and instead listen to a Christian podcast on my drive to work. I think improvising is acceptable, even encouraged. I've also started fasting and praying over specific topics a few mornings per week. My favorite is when I take time to sit on my porch or take a walk to be with God. I alternate between Saturdays and Sundays being a day of rest, and at times I fail to make either work, but it's absolutely worth the intention and effort to try.

Pay attention to the rhythm of your days and weeks, and see where you can be more intentional about time with the Lord. Make a plan to connect consistently with him. Try different ways and different times of the day. I like mornings, but that may not work for you. Journaling, reading devotionals, time in silence and solitude, making art out of bible verses, singing, and listening to worship music are all ways to connect with God. Ask fellow believers how they do this. The only wrong way is not to do it at all. Make time to spend time with your loving Father who loves to spend time with his precious daughter.

Time with Others

I know, I know. I said time spent at church or with other Christians doesn't count as your individual time with God, and I stand by that. What I didn't say is that time in community with other believers is vital. Even though it's not sufficient to help us build intimacy with God, spending time with others is needed for our wellness, and it is part of our calling as Christians.

You might recall the story of Mary and Martha, but I'll summarize the events for you. Jesus came to town and stopped at Martha and Mary's for a visit. Martha wanted to make everything perfect and was busy preparing an amazing meal. Mary wanted to sit at Jesus's feet and absorb every word he spoke. When Martha had enough of doing all the work with no help, she asked Jesus to make her lazy sister get up and help (well, she didn't call her lazy, but I'm pretty sure she thought it). In response to that request Jesus reminded Martha of the most important thing, which was to spend time with him.

This story is usually told with emphasis on being like Mary, at the feet of Jesus, and not being like the busy-body Martha. I'd jump on that train as well, except I think there's more to the story. First, we need others to point us to Jesus and show us how to stop all that we are doing, even the activities that are literally in service to Jesus. We need Marys in our life so we can learn to sit with him in community with others. Second, we also need to serve others. I ask you, how would any Southern Baptist potluck commence without the good-hearted Marthas to bake all those casseroles and pies? The answer is they wouldn't. Community with others means having others to serve you and getting the opportunity to serve others when the time comes. I think we need both Mary and Martha, and we are all called to be like Mary or Martha at one time or another. Martha's mistake wasn't necessarily in being busy serving; it was her failure to recognize the significance of what Mary was doing.

This is one example of the benefit of community. Jesus served with a group of friends. It wasn't always easy, and they disagreed at times about how and when to operate. Some of them even betrayed Jesus in his final hour of need.

Most of us can testify to frustrations with people, perhaps in Christian circles more than others. I'm not sure why that is, perhaps because we expect more of our Jesus-loving friends than others or maybe because Satan wants nothing more than to divide us. I remember very clearly serving with a woman who seemed hell-bent on attacking every single thing I did. It was hurtful and frustrating. Yet I also have been shown so much love by Christian friends. They have shown up, sometimes literally on my front porch, in my hour of need. They have empowered me, encouraged me in my walk, and taught me to be a better wife, mom, and human. They have offered me grace when my behavior was less than graceful and perhaps I was the one being difficult and unkind. I've laughed, cried, and done life with Christian friends, and I treasure that aspect of community more than I loathe the difficulty of some relationships.

If you've got a community, pray about how you can be more invested in it. Look for opportunities to be Martha or Mary. If you don't have community, find one. I realize this isn't always easy; perhaps you've already tried and failed. Try again. Church is a great place for this, and there are plenty of groups and ministries you can join outside of church. I am part of a wonderful women's organization in my community that combines fashion and faith to empower women to be who God created them to be. I'm also part of an online writing community and a member of my local church. I've volunteered with organizations that I've felt called to. These are all groups that are a good fit for me, my interests, and my calling, and they have enriched my life immensely and spurred on my growth in ways that wouldn't have been possible without them. It's also important to be open to allow God to lead you to the right communities. He's full of surprises. Sometimes the best community for you isn't full of people who look like you or share your season of life. Growth is rarely comfortable. Don't write off a community at the first sign of discomfort or in the phase of awkward beginnings. Take your time and give community a chance. Find yours; it's more than worth the effort. And when you do, be engaged and involved. It's nourishing to the soul to feed and be fed by community.

<hr>

Living Out Our Purpose

If this chapter is a recipe for soul nourishment, purpose would be that special ingredient that makes it spectacular. I have lived life without purpose, going from one day to the next. That life can be fulfilling at times, but I've never felt more inspired and full of joy than when I'm walking in my purpose with my God. Take a look back at the chapter on purpose (chapter 6) and try to identify how you can harness this essential ingredient to nourish your soul. God created each of us with a specific purpose in mind, and I've learned it's difficult to be well without walking in purpose and on purpose.

Time with God and time with others will undoubtedly lead you to know and live purposefully. We serve a purposeful God, and he will use our time with him to speak to and nourish our souls, which makes us more prepared to know and live his purpose for us. Being in community gives us opportunity to use our purpose in the body of Christ, each individual contributing uniquely. Many times, I've had friends point out my strengths and encourage me in my purpose, and I've had frequent opportunities to return the favor.

Find ways to nourish your soul by living out your purpose daily. I do this by making time to do little things every day that work toward my purpose. I pray for God to enable me to be purposeful in my work and with my family and friends. I'm not perfect, and I get off track, but each day is a new opportunity to re-engage. I feel like every moment I get to live my purpose is one more sprinkle of that secret ingredient that makes life that much sweeter, and it is abundantly well with my soul.

Sharing Our Story

Living purposefully and being called to a purpose sounds awesome until we bring in vulnerability and start hauling skeletons out of our respective closets. I love to read and hear other people's stories, and I am always inspired when they share the most difficult parts of their lives. When it comes to sharing my own personal journey, I'm not so thrilled. It's hard to be open, especially if it means airing less than flattering dirty laundry. What I've learned when I've been brave enough to be vulnerable is that sharing our story is healing for all souls involved.

Every time I have shared something personal and difficult, there has been at least one person who lets me know how my story helped and encouraged them. In fact, it seems the efficacy of any message is positively correlated with how difficult it was for me to share. I once wrote a blog about grief, sharing my experience with the loss of my father. It was something deeply personal to write, and it felt like I was exposing my heart and soul to the entire world when I hit publish. Then I started to read the responses. People read my gut-wrenching words and were compelled to respond. Some offered compassion and sympathy; others shared how meaningful my words were to their own journey through grief. Had I allowed my reluctance to be vulnerable to stop me from sharing my story, everyone involved would have missed all of that.

Although I share my experiences most often in my writing, I also share in small groups and with friends at times. You don't have to be a writer or have a formal method of sharing your story. Ask God to show you opportunities in your everyday life. Your neighbor or coworker may need to hear what you've gone through. A stranger you strike up a conversation with at the gym or at church may be going through something you've already walked through. Look for opportunities to share, and they'll pop up.

Sharing our story means acknowledging our humanity and inviting the world to share in our experiences. Most of all, it allows Jesus to heal us and use our story to his glory. And all souls in the vicinity who are willing to participate are sure to be individually and collectively nourished.

Gratitude

Last but not least, our souls are nourished by the practice of gratitude. There have been many times I have felt grateful. My wedding day, the day my children were born, the first time my entire family was able to ski on a mountain all together, and the times I get to sit on my porch with a cup of coffee in the quiet of the morning before anyone else rises all come to mind. But life isn't made only of feel-good moments, and neither is my soul. There are peaks and valleys, and sometimes I get sucked into an attitude that is anything but gratitude. When I'm in a valley season, sometimes I forget that even then I should be grateful.

Gratitude is the quickest way I know to go from hopeless to hopeful. When I'm feeling down, I make a list of things I'm grateful for, and this practice has yet to let me down. I put down silly things like my favorite Netflix show or the color red, significant things like the breath in my lungs or people in my life, and spectacular things like the love of a God who loves me even when I'm having a pity party.

Gratitude doesn't always come easily or naturally, though at times it can. Satan loves to help us focus on the negative in our lives and our days, distracting us with despair, guilt, and resentment. Take time to practice regular gratitude. Write down the things you are grateful for, and even share them with the people in your life. When you do, you will literally feel the shift in your soul from suffering to knowing that God is sufficient, faithful, and good.

These five practices, when done consistently, make up a recipe for nourishing our souls. Just like we should exercise, rest, sleep, and feed our bodies to nourish them physically, we need to make regular practice of soul care. Even the healthiest of women physically cannot find true wellness without nurturing their soul. Find small ways in each day to incorporate each of the above, and walk in the wellness God is freely offering to you.

Reflection

1. Consider the five methods of soul nourishment suggested. Which one are you most consistent with? Which one are you needing the most improvement in?
2. How can you ensure you remain consistent in soul nourishing?

3. Plan one thing you can start doing this week to improve in the area you are weakest in. Write a goal here.

11 BECOMING WELL

At the end of any season it's helpful to reflect. As my kids grow up, there are memories I have surprisingly forgotten about until I look at old photos and remember the meaningful moments. True to form, I've taken to writing out our experiences when we go on vacations, because I know in the years to come, I won't remember all the details. Occasionally I get out my vacation memoire and read about our adventures. I'm pleasantly surprised every time I'm reminded of the things we've done and the places we've been.

We've trekked some miles in this journey to wellness, and it's easy to let the seemingly daunting and enormous idea of becoming well overwhelm us to the point of feeling lost and unsure of which direction to take. Before you begin to feel like it's impossible to accomplish all the things outlined in this book, let me release you from the need to do it all and offer instead an opportunity to reflect on your own journey and choose one next step.

Perhaps you've struggled with maintaining motivation, and you need to invest in developing a relationship with Jesus. Spend time with him focusing or refocusing your heart on him and his desires for you. Review the verses, concepts, and questions offered in chapter 2 for help, and trust that the God who is after your heart is more than capable of speaking to and wooing it.

Maybe you're not sure about your identity, worth, and value, and your next step should be to understand those principles in chapter 3, spending time letting those truths soak into your foundational soil, making it fertile ground. We could all use some time revisiting these regularly, reminding us of our identity as daughters of the King, and remembering the worth and value we possess in that identity.

If you've pointed your heart toward Jesus and have absorbed some of his truths, your next step might need to be working on hearing God and blocking out the noise of our intrusive and opinionated world. Develop consistent habits around prayer, reading the Word, and seeking community with the guidance offered in chapter 4.

All of us need healing, and I haven't yet encountered a phase of life when there wasn't a wound or sin I needed to submit in exchange for divine freedom. Your next step might be to prioritize inviting God to reveal what issues are binding you, and chapter 5 can help. There is freedom and beauty to be embraced when we learn to release the things that are weighing us down.

If you've recently experienced a divine removal of your own hackberry trees and have been drawing near to God, growing in your relationship with him, then you are likely learning more about his calling on your life. If that's the case, it's likely your next step should be discovering or rediscovering your purpose. Take a look back at chapter 6 and lean into your purpose, the one God created you to walk out.

If healing from sin, strengthening a spiritual foundation, or exploring purpose aren't your next steps, it's possible you need to identify something in the physical realm. Wherever we are on our wellness journey, the need for physical wellness exists. Chapters 7, 8, and 9 are full of information and inspiration for the well woman to care for her body as the temple it was created to be. The best thing you can do for your overall wellness might be to work on a specific aspect of your physical or mental health.

Finally, if none of those feel like the right step toward your wellness, perhaps it's your soul that is in need of nourishing, and one of the five practices listed in chapter 10 are calling your name.

The truth is, none of us can go wrong by exploring any of the above. The Lord knows what you need to do next, and though I can't tell you which one is the area you should focus on, I can assure you any step you take will be one step closer to walking in the wellness God wants to give you.

I have read about near death experiences and have had a few people share their personal story of seeing heaven in one of these instances. I'll share one story that left me awestruck. This woman had lived through a near death experience and it changed her life. Prior to this experience she lived an unhealthy lifestyle in many ways and ended up undergoing major surgery. It was during this surgery that she found herself in the presence of God, something she could only describe as being freer than she had ever felt before. She wanted so badly to stay in God's peaceful and loving presence but found herself coming back to her earthly life and body. She was initially angry she didn't get to stay in Heaven, but seeing another chance at life on earth she chose to accept her current residency, and do things differently as she waited to return to her real home. Following that heavenly experience, she changed her lifestyle drastically, losing weight and becoming the best version of her earthly self she could possibly become.

Remembering her describe how much better she felt now that she was anticipating her eternal resting place while simultaneously feeling peace in her current physical state, I thought of you and me. This is what I want for us and what I feel God calling us to: anticipating and longing for the day he calls us home while embracing the place he's put us in today. Being intentional about our day-to-day habits and eternal with our focus. Offering ourselves grace when we falter and making better choices when we are given a second chance. Telling others about God's goodness, not because we have to but because we can't stop ourselves. Living this life well, starting today.

Remember the well woman described in the beginning of the book? She's not some fantasy, and her qualities aren't unattainable. In the Book of John there's a story of Jesus having a conversation with a man unable to walk. This man was near a pool of healing waters, awaiting his chance to step into those waters and be healed. When Jesus entered the scene, this guy had been disabled for thirty-eight years. Some of us can relate, as we've been waiting on wellness for what seems like an eternity. The thing is, when Jesus arrived, the wait was over but the calling had just begun, starting with one question. "Do you want to be made well?" Jesus asked (John 5:6 NKJV). This guy, when asked if he wanted the thing he clearly desired more than anything else, didn't respond with an emphatic "Absolutely!" Instead, he started listing the reasons why he hadn't been able to reach the waters, as if Jesus's question was an accusation of laziness and incompetence. I sometimes do the same. When someone offers me release from what's bound me or asks me what I want, suddenly all I can think of is how this world has beaten me up. I want to wallow in the suffering a minute and have someone else recognize what it's been like.

The thing is, Jesus knew the answer before he asked the question, and he saw through the man's lame excuses. Jesus saw everything he had experienced and was ready and waiting to release him from all of that, with one stipulation: he had to take hold of what Jesus was offering. Jesus responded to this man's excuses for illness with instructions for how to step into wellness. He told the man to pick up his mat and walk, and that's precisely what the man did. He took hold of his mat, having faith that this next step held the promise of a wellness he had never known but was suddenly knowable to him through the mere presence of this amazing Savior.

God intends for you to be well, and it's time for you to take hold of this wellness, lay claim to what he's declared for you. Resist the urge to offer excuses or stay on the mat you've become so familiar with. I think Jesus is asking you, like he asked the man in the story, if you want to be made well.

I believe you not only want to be well, you're prepared to do it.

We've covered the material, dug deep into the Word, and equipped ourselves with all manner of information on health and wellness, and it's time for you to pick up your mat and walk as the well woman he already sees you as. Read the description of a well woman again, this time with yourself in mind.

The well woman . . .

Loves the Lord with her whole heart.

Loves others.

Loves herself.

Knows she is a daughter of the King.

Believes she is worthy of being loved.

Knows she is valuable to the Lord.

Acts according to what she knows.

Hears the Lord so loud and clear that the voices of her haters are simply background noise.

Is imperfect and gives her flaws to the Lord.

Is forgiven for her wrongs.

Seeks healing of her wounds and illnesses.

Accepts forgiveness and healing from her loving Father.

Is covered by the righteousness of God, through the gift of Jesus.

Has joy regardless of circumstances.

Is beautiful to behold.

Possesses purpose.

Walks the path God has already laid out for her.

Is uniquely qualified to do what God has put in her path.

Is present and purposeful every day.

Follows through with what the Lord convicts her to do.

Sees her health as both a blessing from and a gift to the Lord.

Commits to daily tasks to seek wellness.

Fills her mind, body, and soul with nourishment.

Allows her physical self to reflect the Holy Spirit inside her.

Bravely displays her scars as her testimony.

Is grateful for the body she has.

Is able.

Is grateful for the life she's been given.

Sees today as a gift.

Knows whose she is and who she is.

She is a well woman.

You are a well woman.

Believe in the goodness of God and his good plans to prosper and not harm you. Believe the things his Word says are true of his children are also true of you. Believe in God's intention and desire for you to be well, and live from this day forward as the well woman you are.

92

NOTES

94

NOTES

96

ABOUT THE AUTHOR

Gena Anderson lives in Central Texas with her husband, Michael, and children Jocelyn and Luke. She can usually be found with her family and dogs, obnoxiously cheering at a kid's sporting event or enjoying the area lakes. She works in Family Medicine at a local clinic, and loves caring for her family and patients. Gena enjoys being active, reading, writing, and traveling. Queso, brownies, and wine are her favorite indulgences, and coffee is simply a requirement for living. Her passion for empowering others to be well is her God-given fuel for daily living. She's thrilled to get the message of this book out into the world.

Website: GenaWrites.com

IG: @GenaAndersonWrites

Other books: No Excuses: a Bible Study on the Book of James
Created Woman Devotional Series 2020
Contributing Author
www.CreatedWoman.net

WHAT'S NEXT?

SUBSCRIBE AND STAY CONNECTED!
Visit GenaWrites.com and subscribe to Well Woman Writing.

Do you want to continue your wellness journey you started with The Well Woman? I send emails regularly with wellness information and inspiration, along with the latest Well Woman events, books, and products. I would love to continue to connect with you and help you experience wellness from here on.

Could you also do me a favor? Leaving a review on Amazon is a gift that takes you only a few minutes but helps an author like me immensely. I would be so grateful for an honest review of this book!

Thank you for reading this book, for sharing it with friends, and for allowing me the honor to speak into your life.

Gena

REFERENCES

[i] Saul McLeod, "Maslow's Hierarchy of Needs," *Simply Psychology,* March 2020, https://www.simplypsychology.org/maslow.html.

[ii] "Facts About Women and Trauma," American Psychological Association, updated August 2017, https://www.apa.org/advocacy/interpersonal-violence/women-traum.

[iii] "Mental Illness," National Institute of Mental Health, updated February 2019, https://www.nimh.nih.gov/health/statistics/mental-illness.shtml.

[iv] "Major Depression," National Institute of Mental Health, updated February 2019, https://www.nimh.nih.gov/health/statistics/major-depression.shtml.

[v] "Any Anxiety Disorder," National Institute of Mental Health, updated November 2017, https://www.nimh.nih.gov/health/statistics/any-anxiety-disorder.shtml.

[vi] "Brain Basics: Understanding Sleep," National Institute of Neurological Disorders and Stroke, updated August 13, 2019, https://www.ninds.nih.gov/Disorders/Patient-Caregiver-Education/Understanding-Sleep.

[vii] Megan Teychenne et al., "Do We Need Physical Activity Guidelines for Mental Health: What Does the Evidence Tell Us?," *Mental Health and Physical Activity*, vol. 18, ScienceDirect.com, March 2020, https://www.sciencedirect.com/science/article/pii/S1755296619301632#bib8.

[viii] J. Thompson Coon et al., "Does Participating in Physical Activity in Outdoor Natural Environments Have a Greater Effect on Physical and Mental Wellbeing Than Physical Activity Indoors? A Systematic Review," *Environmental Science and Technology*, 45 (2011): 1761–72.

[ix] J. K. Garrett et al., "Urban Blue Space and Health and Wellbeing in Hong Kong: Results from a Survey of Older Adults," *Health & Place*, 55 (2019): 100-10.

[x] "Getting Started With Mindfulness," Foundation for a Mindful Society, updated 2020, https://www.mindful.org/meditation/mindfulness-getting-started/.

[xi] M. Manore, "Exercise and the Institute of Medicine's Recommendations for Nutrition," *Current Sports Medicine Reports* 4, (August 4, 2005): 193–98, doi: 10.1097/01.csmr.0000306206.72186.00.